SIRTFOOD DIET

A Beginner's Guide to Fast and Healthy Weight Loss: Lose 7lbs in 7 Days with Easy and Healthy Recipes to Activate the Power of Your Skinny Gene and Burn Fat

By

Danielle T. Clover

© Copyright 2020

All rights reserved.

This report aims to provide accurate and solid data about the point and problem secured. It was possible that the distributor was not obliged to do bookkeeping, formally permitted or otherwise qualified administrations. If an exhortation is relevant, valid or proficient, a rehearsed person should be requested in the call.

The Statement of Standards approved and endorsed by the American Bar Association Committee and the Publishers and Organizations Committee. It is not the least valid in either electronic methods or in a printed community to reproduce, copy or relay some portion of this paper. This delivery is deliberately disallowed, and the report 's capacity is not tolerated unless the distributor's written authorization has been given. All rights held.

The data contained herein is expressed in the sense that any risk, to the extent of absence or otherwise, of any use or abuse of any approaches, procedures or bearings contained in it is a singular, expressive obligation of the beneficiary peruser. No legal liability or responsibility would be taken against the seller for any fix, damage, or money-related misfortune due to the data in this regard, either explicitly or impliedly.Special creators claim all copyrights that the seller does not have.The details herein are only provided for instructional purposes and are all-inclusive. The details were reached without a document or other guarantee of security.The marks used shall be without consent, and the mark shall be distributed without the consent or support of the proprietor. All trademarks in this book are solely for explanation and are clearly owned by the owners not associated with this record.

TABLE OF CONTENTS

INTRODUCTION

The Sirtfood diet, which was first introduced in 2016, remains a popular subject and involves people following a diet high in "sirt-foods." According to the food authors, these unique foods function by stimulating certain proteins called sirtuins in the body. Sirtuins are believed to defend the cells of the body from dying while under tension and to regulate inflammation, metabolism and the ageing cycle. The sirtuins are believed to influence the body's capacity to lose fat and improve the metabolism, producing a weight reduction of seven pounds a week while maintaining muscle. Many researchers suggest that it is impossible for this to simply be a fat reduction, but rather represents improvements in skeletal muscle and hepatitis glycogen stocks.

The Sirtfood Diet is the latest means of quickly shifting weight without drastic diet by triggering the same 'skinny gene' pathways normally done only with exercise and fasting. Some foods contain chemicals called polyphenols which stress our cells mildly and which turn on genes that imitate the effects of fasting and exercise. The sirtuin pathways that influence metabolism, ageing and mood are activated by food rich in polyphenols – like broccoli, dark chocolate and red wine. A diet rich in this Sirtfood kicks off weight loss while maintaining optimum health, without sacrificing muscle.

Add healthy Sirt foods to your diet to reduce your weight, gain incredible energy and vibrant health effectively and sustainably. Switch your corporeal fat-burning forces, weight loss overcharging and help stave disease off with this easy-to-follow diet developed by nutritional experts who have demonstrated the impact of Sirt foods. Dark chocolate, coffee, kale – all of them are foods which cause sirtuins and turn on what is known as 'skinny genes' in your body. The Sirtfood Diet offers you a simple, healthy way of eating for the loss of weight, delicious easy-to-use recipes and a long-term success maintenance plan. The Sirtfood Diet is a non-exclusion lifestyle, and Sirt foods are readily accessible and inexpensive. This is a lifestyle that allows you to appreciate savory, nutritious food and the effects of weight loss while taking your knife at weight bifurcation.

The program explains that consuming these foods would trigger the "skinny gene" route, and you will lose seven kilograms in seven days. Foods, including spinach, dark chocolate, and wine contain a natural chemical called polyphenol, which imitate fitness and fasting results. Fresh mango, red onions, cinnamon and turmeric, are also good Sirt foods. These foods stimulate the path of sirtuin to induce weight loss. Science sounds appealing, but there is no evidence to support such arguments. Moreover, the expected weight loss pace in the first week is relatively high and does not align with the National Institute for Health's recommendations on healthy weight loss of one to two pounds a week.

WHAT IS THE SIRT FOOD

The appearance of a fictional science snack is actually a food spike in sirtuin activators, according to nutritionist Rob Hobson. Sirtuins are a form of protein which protects the cell in our bodies from death or disease, but also, work has shown that they help to control metabolism, increase muscle levels and improve fat loss – the current name "Wonder Food."

The Sirtfood Diet has been established by two prominent nutritionists working for a private gym in the UK.

Who came up with the Sirtfood Diet?

A pair of writers and wellness experts, Aidan Goggins and Glen Matten, have also concentrated on good health rather than lack of weight. The Sirtfood Diet's latest book contains three Sirtfood green juices per day, followed by nutritious meals, such as buckwheat and crept stir-fry or smoked salmon super salad.

What can you eat on the Sirtfood Diet?

The Sirt Food Diet plan focuses on adding healthy Sirt food to your intake. These are as follows:

- Red wine
- Apples
- Citrus fruits
- Dark chocolate
- Buckwheat
- Walnuts
- Capers
- Medjool dates
- Parsley
- Soy
- Blueberries
- Green tea
- Strawberries
- Olive oil
- Turmeric
- Rocket
- Kale.

Interestingly, another highlight is coffee, which is very welcome news if you are in love with caffeine. Countries that already eat a high amount of Sirt foods include Japan and Italy, both regularly ranked among the healthiest countries in the world.

Phases of the diet

The diet comprises of two phases; the initial one-week duration comprises of calories being limited to 1000 kcal for three days with a normal intake of three Sirtfood green juices and one Sirtfood-rich meal. The juice contains kale, celery, rocket, Persil, green tea and citrus fruit. The food contains turkey with garlic, cabers and parsley, chicken and kale curry and creeping filled with noodles of buckwheat. Intakes from four to seven days are raised to 1500kcal, consisting of two Sirt-food green juices and two meals rich in Sirtfood per day.

Although the diet promotes healthy foods, it is restrictive in food choices as well as daily calories, particularly in the initial stages. It also includes consuming water, which meets the present normal requirements during Step one.

The second phase is referred to as the 14-day maintenance phase, where steady weight loss takes place. The writers think it's a permanent and practical method of reducing weight. However, weight reduction is not the objective of the diet – it is intended for consuming the best food that nature has to bring. They recommend three balanced Sirt foods rich with one green Sirt food juice per day.

Getting Started

The Sirtfood Diet includes regular juices. Make sure you've got a juicer. Three primary ingredients are also required.

Matcha is a powdered green tea and an important green juice ingredient. It is easily accessible online if it is not kept at the nearest health food shop. Likewise, lovage, a herb in the green juice recipe, may sometimes seem difficult to find. But seeds can easily be bought online to grow in a pot as a plant.

Buckwheat, finally. It's a great substitute to more traditional grains, but most supermarkets mix their buckwheat items with wheat. In your nearest organic food shop, you are more likely to find 100% buckwheat.

Meal Ideas

For breakfast, try soy milk, blended fruit, sliced walnuts and dark chocolate, an omelet filled with bacon, red chicory, and parsley for the savory.

The Sirt food salad is perfect for lunch – but a wholemeal pitta with meat, cheese, or hummus, whether you like any carbohydrates, is nutritious and soothing.

Dinner time must not be boring, either: stir-fried crew with kale noodles and buckwheat is a perfect dinner at night. And, believe it or not, though it's the way of Sirt food, pizza is still on the menu.

Is there a Sirtfood Diet plan?

Yes, there is. Here's what it looks like:

Week 1:

- Limit your consumption to one thousand calories a day.
- Consume three Sirt-food green juices in a day.
- Enjoy one Sirt-food rich meal a day.

Week 2:

- Up to 1500 calories a day.
- Consume two Sirt-food green juices a day.
- Enjoy two Sirt-food high-quality meals a day.

There is no fixed plan in the long run. It is all about adjusting your lifestyle to the maximum number of Sirt foods that should make you feel healthier and energetic.

Who follows the Sirtfood Diet already?

Adele, Jodie Kidd, Lorraine Pascale and Sir Ben Ainslie are already part of the growing celebrity fans of the Sirtfood Diet.

Is It Effective?

Sirtfood Diet overwhelms weight loss, transforms the "skinny gene," and avoids diseases.

The problem is that there is no research to back it up. Till date, there is no compelling proof that the Sirt-food Diet is more effective than other calorie-restricted diets for weight loss.

And while all of these products have medicinal properties, no long-term human trials have been conducted to figure out whether Sirt-food rich diets provide measurable health benefits. The Sirt-food Diet book, however, reports the results of a pilot study carried out by the authors involving 39 gym participants. However, it seems that the findings of this analysis have not been published elsewhere.

The patients observed the diet for a week and practiced every day. At the end of the week, average participants lost 7 pounds (3.2 kg) and maintained or even gained muscle mass. The reduction of calorie consumption to 1,000 calories and regular workout nearly can invariably contribute to weight loss.

However, such a fast weight reduction is neither real nor long-lasting, so subjects were not tracked by this analysis beyond the first week to see whether they managed to regain the weight, as is usually the case.

In addition to consuming fat and tissue, the body utilizes emergency energy reserves of glycogen. Each glycogen molecule needs 3–4 water molecules to be processed. When the body uses glycogen, this water is always extracted. It is termed "water weight." Only about a third of the weight reduction is extracted from fat during the first week with severe calorie limits, whereas the remaining two-thirds is generated from the skin, muscle and glycogen. When the calorie consumption rises, the body fills its glycogen reserves, and the weight returns.

Unfortunately, this form of calorie restriction can even decrease the body's metabolic rate, which implies that you need to consume much fewer calories each day. This diet will probably help you lose a couple of pounds at first, but it will probably return once the diet has ended.

Three weeks are, therefore, not long enough for it to have a meaningful long-term effect on disease prevention.

On the other hand, it may be a smart idea to introduce Sirt food to your daily diet in the long run. But in this situation, you may also miss the diet and continue to do so. This diet will help you lose weight since it is low in calories, so it is possible the weight will increase after the diet finishes. The diet is too short to have a long-term health effect.

HOW TO FOLLOW THE SIRTFOOD DIET

The Sirtfood Diet continues for a minimum of three weeks in two stages. You will then proceed to "certify" your diet by using as many Sirt foods as you can in your meals. In The Sirtfood Diet book, written by the diet's creators, the specific recipes for these two phases are presented. The meals are filled with Sirt foods which contain other components in addition to the "max 20 Sirtfoods." Nonetheless, three of the necessary signature ingredients — matcha green tea powder, lovage and buckwheat — may be costly or hard to recognize.

A big aspect of the diet is green tea, which you will create two or three times a day. A juicer (a blender doesn't work) and a kitchen scale are required, as the weight of the ingredients are provided. Here is the recipe:

- 75 grams (2.5 oz) kale
- 30 grams (1 oz) arugula (rocket)
- Sirtfood Green Juice
- Two celery sticks
- 5 grams parsley
- 1 cm (0.5 in) ginger
- half a lemon

- half a green apple
- half a teaspoon matcha green tea powder

Mix all the ingredients and put them into a bowl. Pick the lemon by then, then mix in the water both the lemon juice and the green tea powder.

Phase One

Step one lasts seven days and requires minimal calories and lots of green tea. This helps you start your weight loss while claiming to help you lose 7 pounds (3.2 kg) in seven days.

The calorie intake during the first three days of phase one is limited to 1,000 calories. You should consume three green juices a day plus one breakfast. Every day you can choose from the book's recipes, which all include sirt-food as the main component of the meal.

Food sources are miso-glazed tofu, Sirtfood omelet, or buckwheat stir-fry shrimp.

Days 4–7 of step one boost the calorie consumption to 1,500. This includes two green juices a day and two additional Sirt foods that you can choose from the book.

Phase Two

The second process lasts two weeks. You will continue to lose weight throughout this "maintenance" process.

For this phase, there is no specific calorie limit. Instead, three Sirtfood meals and one green juice a day are offered. Again, the food is picked from the book's recipes.

After the Diet

These two steps can be replicated as much as you like for more weight reduction. However, during these stages, you are advised to try to "certify" your diet by including Sirt-foods daily in your meals.

There are a variety of Sirtfood Diet books filled with Sirt-food recipes. Also, as a snack or in recipes you already use, you should have Sirt food. You are often advised to drink green tea on a regular basis.

This makes the Sirtfood Diet more of a change in lifestyle than a one-time diet.

Is Sirtfoods the New Superfoods?

Nobody disputes that Sirtfood is perfect for you. Their nutrients are often high, and they are full of healthy plant compounds. In fact, many of the items prescribed for the Sirtfood Diet have been correlated with health benefits.

For example, a moderate intake of dark chocolate with a high level of cocoa can reduce the risk of heart disease and help combat inflammation. Green tea can decrease the risk of stroke and diabetes and reduce blood pressure.

And turmeric has anti-inflammatory effects which generally benefit the body and can even protect against chronic inflammatory diseases.

Indeed, most Sirtfoods have shown health benefits in humans. However, there is preliminary evidence for the health benefits of raising the levels of a sirtuin protein. However, animal and cell work has generated promising outcomes.

Researchers have found, for example, that elevated sirtuin protein levels lead to a longer life for yeast, worms and mice.

Sirtuin proteins tell the body to burn greater fat for energy during fasting or calorie limitations and improve insulin sensitivity. In one study in a mouse, increased sirtuin levels resulted in fat loss. Some evidence suggests that sirtuins can also help to reduce inflammation, prevent tumor development and delay heart disease, as well as Alzheimer's progress.

Although experiments in mice and human cells have shown positive results, no human studies have investigated the effects of increased sirtuin rates. Consequently, it is not clear that increased levels of sirtuin protein in the body contribute to longer lifetimes or lower cancer risks in humans.

Work is currently underway to produce compounds that raise the number of sirtuins in the body efficiently. Human research will, therefore, begin to explore the impact of sirtuins on human safety. Before then, the consequences of elevated sirtuin rates cannot be calculated.

Is It Healthy and Sustainable?

Almost all Sirt foods are safe options and may also provide safety advantages because of their antioxidant or anti-inflammatory effects. However, consuming a few especially nutritious foods can not satisfy the dietary needs in the body.

The Sirtfood Diet is overly restrictive and does not deliver obvious, special health benefits over any other diet. In fact, consuming only 1000 calories are typically not prescribed without a doctor's supervision. Even 1,500 calories a day is too limiting for certain people to consume.

The diet always requires one to drink up to three natural juices a day. Although juices can be a good source of vitamins and minerals, they contain virtually no safe fibers, like entire fruits and vegetables.

In fact, drinking tea all day long is a terrible thing for both your blood sugar and your teeth. Not to mention, since the diet is so limited in calories and dietary choices, including protein, vitamins and minerals are more than likely deficient, particularly in the first phase.

This diet can be difficult to stick to for the whole three weeks due to the low calorie and the restrictive dietary choices.

In addition to the initial high costs of purchasing a juicer, books and other unusual and expensive products and the time it requires to cook different meals and drinks, this lifestyle has become impractical for certain people and wasteful.

Safety and Side Effects

While the first step in the Sirtfood Diet is very low in calories and nutritionally incomplete, a typically active person may not have any major safety issues, given the limited length of the diet.

However, for people with diabetes, calorie restriction and consuming only juice for the first few days of their diet can contribute to dangerous blood sugar changes. However, a stable person can also have certain side effects — primarily malnutrition.

Eat just 1,000–1,500 calories a day, and almost anyone would feel hungry, particularly if you drink juice which is low in fiber, a nutrient that should make you feel whole.

Many negative effects, such as weakness, lightheadedness and irritability, may arise during stage one as a result of calorie restriction.

Serious health consequences for an otherwise healthy adult are unlikely if the diet is followed for just three weeks. The Sirtfood Diet is made of nutritious foods but is not necessarily safe.

Its theory and health claims are based, not to mention, on major extrapolations from preliminary scientific evidence. Although it is not a terrible thing to attach certain Sirt foods to your diet, and which may also have health benefits, the diet itself seems like just another fad.

Increase food resources now to create good, long-term lifestyle improvements.

THE HEALTH BENEFITS

There is proof that sirtuin activators may provide a wide variety of health benefits as well as muscle strengthening and appetite suppression. That involves having better memory, better control of blood sugar levels in the body, and the clearance of damage caused by free radical molecules that build up in cells and result in cancer and other diseases.

"The positive effects of the intake of food and beverages rich in sirtuin activators in decreasing chronic disease risk are important observational evidence," said Professor Frank Hu, an authority on diet and epidemiology at Harvard University in a recent paper in Advances In Nutrition. An anti-ageing diet is particularly suited to a Sirt food diet.

While the entire plant realm is home to sirtuin activators, only some fruits and vegetables have enough to report as Sirtfood. Examples include green tea, cacao powder, Indian spice pea, spinach, onion and parsley.

In many stores, fruit and vegetables such as strawberries, avocados, bananas, spinach, kiwis, broccoli, and pep are actually quite low activators for sirtuins. This does not mean, however, that they are not worth eating because they have many other advantages.

The advantage of a Sirtfood-packed diet is that it's much more versatile than other diets. You could just consume a few Sirt foods healthily. Or you could concentrate on them. The 5:2 diet could require more calories on low-calorie days by incorporating Sirt foods.

One notable observation of a Sirtfood diet trial is that participants lose excessive weight without weakening their muscles. It was also normal for participants to build weight, contributing to a more formed and toned body. It is the beauty of Sirtfoods: fat burning is activated, but muscle growth, maintenance and repair are promoted as well. In comparison to other foods, weight reduction typically occurs from fat and muscle, which slows down the digestion of the body and allows weight to rebound more easily.

Are there any other benefits of Sirtfoods?

Sirtuins have a hand in several other safe advantages as well. Including:

Sleep Activating sirtuins adds to improving of the circadian cycle such that you generate hormones while you improve your sleep cycle.

Diabetes

Sirtuins allow cells to be more responsive to insulin so that they can lose more blood glucose. As the key to both diabetes and weight gain is insulin resistance, there can be positive news for the waistline.

Memory

Turmeric boosts short-term performance and defends against cognitive disorders. Pack your morning juice to begin the day more brainy.

LEAN GENE

Genetics is a long-standing beat-up cause. This is why people are lazy, weak, and behave as though they do not realize what's going on in their lives. Yeah, certain mutations may render you predisposed to a disease, but that does not indicate that must have it as you get older. You can also ensure that you grow good genes in life by not building poor habits. It means that you can build as strong an atmosphere as you can to prevent inherited vulnerabilities.

It appears like biology is the direction in which our scientific world shifts. This is terrifying. Essentially, our chromosomes are what creates us. If we fix the right genetic code somewhere, we could all be the same. There has been a lot of talk about tests in mice and the consequences of "obesity mutation." They want to see why people are fat.

The obesity gene was long known, but just recently, how this gene functions was revealed. We named the FTO mutation, and mice who had not pigged the mutation were slouched all day long and miraculously appeared more healthy. It seems like the right cure for individuals to do or feed properly. Any other study has shown that individuals with this amazing FTO gene have an excess of 7 pounds heavier and 70% more likely to be obese. 70% is a big amount.

Either we have individuals who will not want to remain alive, or this gene is just an end to all genes. My guess is that people don't want to remain safe.

Mice are really similar to us when it comes to our genes and DNA, and the experiments performed on this mouse will demonstrate how we accumulate any extra weight from this FTO mutation. To pharmaceutical firms, this is a fairly major move. Their number has projected about 400 million obese people in the world and its rising. Here in states, for every three men, 2 of them are overweight. These figures are bad, but they get worse. This indicates that something about the program is incorrect. All this needs to be changed.

Being obese raises any risk factor that you could think about. If you have to bear this additional weight, your body faces a lot more pain than normal. Imagine wearing a dumbbell weighing around 50 pounds anywhere you go.

Such studies will ultimately contribute to obesity care. They view obesity as a disorder and not as a preference for lifestyle. People may lose weight; the FTO gene may or may not be lost. Some will consider it difficult, but it is always feasible. I can see the future. I will see the future. When the first advert on television speaks about the consequences of the FTO mutation, they inquire if you are fat with certain alarming figures, then comes the main selling advertisement on whatever the medication is.

This is my pet peeve. Why do we investigate this? Yeah, for the sake of information, it is necessary and can be achieved, but why not look to the past where the citizens were not fat? See how slim they were, what they were drinking and how they were sleeping. We will avoid researching illness here in pursuit of wellness—health research to determine fitness. Look at mature cultures that were generally healthy. Look at how strong and slim they were.

So, my aim is to avoid researching illness in order to pursue wellness. Do not allow your chromosomes to dictate who you are and how you are. Your climate and biology play an important role, and I think it plays a more important role than we think. You have the opportunity to improve yourself, whether it be autism, a professional athlete, succeeding in school or some other reason. You should do it, whether it's healthy genes or not.

Do You Have Lean Genes?

What is your genetic weight? Just 5% of all weight disorders compensate for obesity genes. About 95% of the weight issues are due to chromosomes. This fact has not affected our culture's high incidence of obesity. Nor should we blame the issue of obesity on high-fat diets. Because fat contains nine calories per gram, unlike the carbs or protein that only contain four calories per gram, our crisis still cannot be nailed to fat consumption. Evidence has demonstrated, in addition, that low-fat diets do not work well and do more damage than good. And to add to that –avoiding fat in your diet is not a major determinant of body fat. The Women's Wellness Project, the first diet and body weight research study, showed that 50,000 people have no substantial loss of weight in low-fat diets.

Were you conscious that you may potentially be at an "ideal" weight that looks fine and in knowingly severely obese? We refer to it as "Skinny Fat." Many models who you find to be slim or lean may potentially have a large proportion of body fat. Anything higher than 30% is clinically obese. Some of these "ideal" images have very little lean mass on their frames. As we always claim, they are simply just skin and bones, and we must often have fat under the skin in our definition. This is really important to learn what the real body fat or muscle fat percentage is. This marker determines not only your real slimness but also your actual health. That is why I still suggest that you check your body fat composition.

But without the specific check – the main way to avoid slipping into the 'skinny-fat' group is a full and healthy diet. Here's a trick - because you have a higher rating, you will consume better. Meaning, if you have more lean muscle mass than fat to sustain your weight, you will potentially consume more. Your body is a robotic oven that can break down everything you consume quickly – and comfortably. Not that it all burns down quickly. If you consume unhealthy foods into your body, your muscle mass reduces, and the capacity to lose calories is therefore reduced. There are two main things that improve lean muscle mass - exercise resistance and protein. Both inappropriate proportions for your body type and your workout intensity should give you the perfect fat - lean muscle ratio.

Turning to the topic of obesity and weight care, the main aspect is to personalize the strategy. We learn more and more about something named Nutri-genomics in my area of agriculture. It is the awareness of how we can affect our genes through food. Yeah, this has been learned - our diet will affect and probably alter the expression of our genome. If you like, let's name it Genetic Eating. When we supply the body with building blocks and good nutrients, the genes "turn on" as it were. Put simply - you come into this world with some genetic make-up, and if you do not properly "feed" your genes-the healthy expression of those genes are stopped. For example, let us refer to it as the "good weight gene" without the proper nutrients, this gene shuts down. To switch the genetic light on, we will need to send our body the correct current (a little wordplay) – for it to work.

This is, in reality, a very basic description for a very complicated operation. The most important aspect you can realize is that you should adjust your DNA to blend in with your clothes, so YOUR Food is one of the most important functions.

A SIRTFOOD DIET MEAL PLAN

It is described as the kilo-shredding program in which you are encouraged to drink chocolate and red wine and are promised to be like a supermodel and a superhero.

In Instagram, it's the stuff UFC featherweight king Conor McGregor does. A few days before his first two big 2016 matches against Nate Diaz, the Irishman took a selfie - and it was liked by over 116,000 users.

This's what Adele and Jodie Kidd are doing – so for naysayers, of course, it's just the new fad, another calorie restricting scheme that creates claims that can't be held to.

But the fact is, behind Sirt there is much more scientific influence than the usual drop-fat quick scheme. It is based on a class of compounds discovered over the last decade, and recent data shows they are far more significant than commonly believed. So if the people behind it are correct, we have to turn our attention to what we consume.

Is the Sirt Diet Just Another Fad?

What's the evidence? And what's the science behind it all?

The science, first of all, is this. A community of Silent Knowledge Regulator (SIR) proteins – named after Sirt – are proteins that ramp up our metabolism, improve muscle performance, trigger fat burning processes, minimize inflammation and remedy cell damage. Simply put, sirtuins make us safer, more healthy and are mild (there is also proof that they can help battle severe problems like Alzheimer's disease and diabetes, and moreso at noon).

Mild forms of stress – including exercise and calory limitation – trigger the body's sirtuin production, but recent discoveries have found that chemicals known in fruit and vegetables as sirtuin activators can do the same. Some foods – Sirt foods as called by diet makers Aidan Goggins and Glen Matten – are especially high in those sirtuin activators. And so the theory is that you will lose fat and improve your health when eating a diet made up of those foods.

Goggins and Matten created the Sirt Plan, the 7-day meal program, to check the theory. It is easy: the regular intake of calories for the first three days is reduced to 1.000 and consists of three grassy juices and a meal rich in Sirtfood. The consumption of calories is raised to 1.500 on days four to seven and is composed of two drinks and two meals. After the first week, a healthy diet full of Sirt foods and more green juices would be prescribed. This sounds terrible on the surface: even most quick diets give more calories. However, is it?

Rannoch Donald, a coach and teacher who pursued the diet, says: "I felt it all challenging. "The juice is essential: it's like the fuel of a rocket. The first week was accompanied by easy sailing, during which I was 5 kg lighter for three weeks. But more notably, in a few years, I thought the strongest I ever had. I was reducing my body weight; I was happier eating; I didn't have any issues with the body; I felt healthy, I was studying, practicing, and fantastically dealing with a half dozen lessons a week from even the most horrible session in Brazil."

Goggins and Matten hired 37 people from XK Gym, including 15 overweight, to check the diet in a broader context. All of these workouts were mild, none were thorough, and only some continued to do fewer. And the test results were surprising after just one week, even with the calorie limitation: the participants lost a total of 3 kg of weight but instead placed on only 0.8 kg of muscle. You should hope to lose an average of 1 kg from a normal diet that lowers the calories in a week to the same amount.

Why is Sirt not available?

There is the obvious question: if sirtuins improve so much, why aren't pharmaceutical firms rushing to pill it into a type of supplement? Short reply: since they still do not grasp the process by which they function entirely, their materials would not always be as easily consumed by the body as the normal types.

Goggins and Matten point to the resveratrol example. In fact, its absorption by the body is low, but its bioavailability (How much the body can use) is at least six times higher than its natural food matrix of red wine. We agree that it's healthier to consume a large variety of such nutrients in the form of natural whole-foods that coexist with the hundreds of other bioactive chemical plants, which function in a synergistic manner to improve our wellbeing.

Fast and furious?

This is, of course, the part of the sirt-diet which is criticized. Usually, the program relies in the early stages on calorie restriction, at least, and the weight reduction of more than 1 kg a week is, according to prior practice, unsafe or unrealistic. This is a legitimate concern: early lack of calories appears to come from calorie depletion and reduced water fluctuation in the majority of diets for calories and, as recently studied by participants in The Biggest Loser reveals, rationing yourself will slow your metabolism down every day to an almost permanent crawl.

But that's not what Sirt does, Goggins and Matten answer. Yeah, the diet represents certain facets of fasting, and Sirt-foods tend to turbo-charge the impact of a calorie limit for the first seven days of the maximum diet. But it's a little tougher than looking for short-term improvements. And how does that work? Why does it work? Ok, firstly, the "energy" part of the equation must be grasped. "Everyone in their lives needs a certain amount of stress," says Goggins. "We build tension on the body every time we exercise, which can be a positive or a negative thing. There are temptations to still work hard, to strive harder. However, this carries the risk of excessively stressed growth; as well as the risk of burnout and weakening immune systems. "On the other hand: you can improve the capacity of the body to deal with higher rates of stress while being subjected to higher levels of stress. "Animal stress reactions are probably more developed than our own," Goggins says. "Think about it: we can go to the hungry and thirsty for food and drink; we consider shade too hot; we run from assaults. The plants, on the other hand, are stagnant and must tolerate many of these physiological pressures and risks. Over the past billions of years, they have therefore built a highly sophisticated stress response mechanism that humiliates [human beings], creating an enormous array of natural vegetable chemical products – called polyphenols – that allows them to adjust and thrive effectively to their climate. When we eat these plants, we eat the nutrients of polyphenols, which cause our own inherent mechanisms of stress reaction. We are talking almost the same path as fasting and exercising – sirtuins." According to Goggins, polyphenols are the one item that the traditional American diet has plenty of, so when excluded from the diet, the much-valued Mediterranean diet lacks almost complete efficacy. Via mermaids, polyphenols may be used to imitate Brown Adipose tissue ("good" fat that helps to produce body heat) across a variety of weight loss results, including promoting white adipose tissue (traditionally poor fat). They also assist with stomach satisfaction problems by increasing the response of the body to the satiety hormone leptin.

"These natural plant compounds are often labelled 'calorie-restrictive mimetic' as they can alter the beneficial results of fasting in our cells, such as fat burning," says Goggins. "The results are shifting the game. Although we have more sophisticated signaling molecules than our own, the effects are comparable to what we would do alone."

The real health foods

Sirt often has more nutrients than the makeup of the bone. In addition to the experiments by Goggins and Matten, more scientifically monitored studies on Sirtfoods yielded positive performance. In October 2015, for example, Columbia University researchers in New York noticed the dissolution of drinking water in 19 intermediate-age topics with a gram of cacao, particularly rich in sirtuin-enhanced epicatechin.

In November of the same year, Monash University researchers in Melbourne recorded that, if patients in the early phases of type 2 diabetes applied a gram of turmeric a day to their diets, their working memory increased. There are some indications for diabetics that sirtuin activation raises the volume of insulin that can be secreted and makes it function more efficiently. In the skeleton, sirtuins promote osteoblast growth and preservation, a cell group responsible for the formation of new bones.

When more work is carried out, the next big thing for Sirt will be its connection to leucine, the leading muscle builder in the branched-chain amino acids (BCAAs). Leucine is a main protein synthesis regulator and stimulates a protein called mTOR (although you don't have to think about it to grasp the next bit).

"Leucine is a blade with two sides," Goggins says. "It's a muscle accelerator, but if you don't have the internal machines to handle it, the engine will explode." Theoretically, having a more Sirt food heavy diet can increase your body's protein content so that it can successfully absorb the old recommendation of "20-30 g a sitting" in the past.

All this, of course, needs further work. Thirty-seven participants in one research gym and other experiments on the effect of sirtuins on animals or human cells have been performed – and neither expected to accurately reflect what occurs inside the body. But despite all skepticism of the more extreme arguments of food, by adopting a variant of the Sirt Plan, it is difficult to see what you are to sacrifice. Although you would not put up the calorie-limited version of the diet and go right into the "maintenance" phase. In the so-called Blue Zones, places of the world such as Sardinia and Okinawa, where people live longer and healthier lives, you would have eaten a wide variety of foods.

"I don't like the word diet, so this is a lifestyle plan rather than a quick-fire operation," Donald says. "It's just healthy living. Yet, with the introduction of green juice cocktails, the general approach remains to integrate balanced whole-of-life products rather than to deify 'superfoods'." Or, to put it another way: you won't get happier unless more spinach, tomatoes, walnuts or red wine are introduced. Particularly if you're not a UFC or a supermodel fighter.

The Meal Plan

With these values, here's what should be on the menu during the maintenance process over a week (green juices aside).

Breakfast:

- Fruit smoothie made with rolled oats and soy milk
- Kale omelet
- Muesli, yoghurt and blueberries

Lunch and dinner:

- Rocket salad with tuna, tomatoes and cucumber dressed in olive oil
- Grilled fish with buckwheat salad
- Veggie-packed spicy tofu stir fry with birds-eye chili
- Chicken and soba noodle stir fry
- Kale salad with edamame beans and red onion dressed in olive oil
- Tofu burgers with wholegrain bread and salad
- Spicy chicken curry served with wholegrain brown rice

Snacks:

- Walnuts

- Coffee

- Celery and hummus

- Dark chocolate

- Fresh fruit, particularly strawberries, apples and oranges

WHAT ARE THE BLUE ZONES

The Dan Buettner National Geographic Fellow outlines the most popular food, nutrition and lifestyle patterns from the Blue Zones, which are geo-cultural zones around the globe where the longest living people are known to stay. The blue areas include extraordinarily large rates of decades of age and lifespan, aged well over a century without any diseases like heart failure, obesity, cancer or diabetes.

It consists of Ikaria, Greece; Okinawa, Japan; Sardinia's Ogliastra region; Loma Linda, California (but only the greater 7th Day Adventist community); and Costa Rica's the Nicoya Peninsula.

Five recognized Blue Zones are defined by Buettner:

1. **Icaria, Greece:** This Greek island is closer than anything in the world to the Mediterranean diet. The citizens here live almost seven years longer than the average Americans — and around a quarter of the disease epidemics affect them. And, get this: among Icarians over 80 years old, almost nine out of ten people and seven out of the ten women still walk every day (compared with one out of two men and one out of four women in the rest of Greece), a studio from Athens, Greece, reports.

2. **Ogliastra, Sardinia (Italy):** The Italian island is host to the world's greatest concentration of centuries-old people. They are mainly shepherds in 14 communities, remaining busy throughout their lives and consuming a predominantly vegetable diet along with pork and red wine.

3. **Okinawa, Japan:** The oldest people in the world reside in this archipelago, in reality, certain areas of the land have 30 times more female centenarians per capita than in the United States. Its sustainability is grounded in good social networks and diets focused on vegetables.

4. **Nicoya, Costa Rica:** People in this city in the central peninsula are above three times more likely (and healthy) to hit 90 than more Americans. Moreover, the lowest risk of middle-aged mortality in the world is in this region of Costa Rica (think less heart failure and diabetes). The Nicoya diet is focused on breasts, maize tortillas and culture that holds physical activity as an ancient part. And, the Nicoyans have a sense of existence (another distinctive characteristic of the Blue Zones), which they term the "plan de Vida."

5. **Loma Linda, California**: Surprised America's on the list? This zone is unique to the 7th day Adventists who have shunned sugar, dairy, food, cigarettes and, sometimes, coffee drinks and eat based on a healthier diet and exercise, a religious minority centered in the suburb of San Bernardino.

Food Choices for Longevity

None of the centenarians of the Blue Zones I've ever known attempted to survive to 100. At 50, nobody said, "You know what, I'm going to stay on this longevity diet and live another 50 years!" They don't count calories, minerals or even read packets, or measure protein grams. They do not restrict their consumption of food — in reality, all of them rejoice with food. As we have used the experience of the world diet for the regeneration of cities in the United States, I have come to feel that we will build the same kind of community here.

It starts with choices of food. Most of the Blue Zones' residents that I have encountered have good access to local fruits and vegetables, mostly free of pesticides and organically cultivated. If such foodstuffs are not produced in their own farms, it is feasible for them to buy them and they are more economical than refined alternatives.

They also choose some healthy items for their regular or weekly meals — foods frequently not seen either in grocery stores or on quick food menus in the nation. They have acquired recipes or created recipes for themselves in order to try nutritious foods — a big aspect of the Blue Zones lifestyle, and if you don't enjoy what you consume, you won't eat them for too long.

The specific foods that are essential to centuries-old Blue Zones differ from one culture to another. However, the food selection recommendations which we formulated after visits to various blue zones, and the best way to translate these values for North Americans, could be just as relevant.

The outcomes are a long-term, systematic and empirical analysis. We wanted the knowledge that was not only factual or focused on observations, kitchen visits or dinners with a hundred-year-old. We examined over 150 nutritional experiments over the last century from Blue Zones and then condensed these research to a worldwide snapshot of what people hundreds of years in age actually eat.

Here are a few recommendations you should adopt to consume the diet.

BLUE ZONES FOOD GUIDELINES

Employ these recommendations, and you can evict processed food starches and carbohydrates, replacing them with balanced, nutrient-dense and fiber-rich ingredients — and do it naturally.

1. Plant Slant: See that 95% of the food comes from one or more plants

Limit animal protein to just one limited portion a day in your diet. Take preference to vegetables, plants, yams, pies, bananas, nuts and seeds. Whole grains are all right too. Although people consume meat in four of the five Blue Areas, they consume it sparingly, as a meal, as a tiny side, or as a way to sample beef.

"Food is like plutonium, and we don't know how healthy it is," as our advisor Walter Willett from the Harvard School of Public Health puts it. In fact, research suggests that vegetarian Adventists of 30 years of age are likely to survive their meat consuming peers by eight years. At the same time, the amount of natural products in your meals has several beneficial results. In the Blue Areas, while they are in the season, people consume a number of garden plants and either wine or dry the surplus in the off-season.

Leafy greens such as spinach, coffee, beet and turbot tops, chard and collards are among the best long-life foods available in the Blue Zone diet. More than 75 varieties of foodstuffs emerge like weeds in Ikaria; many produce ten times the polyphenols present in red wine. Studies have shown that in the next four years, people who consume the average of a cup of cooked greens are twice as likely to die as those who did not eat vegetables.

Researchers also found that those who eat a quarter of a pound of fruit every day (roughly an apple) are 60% less likely to die in the next four years than those who did not. Most oils come from animals, so all of them are safer than animal fats. We cannot assume that olive oil is the only good plant oil, but it is the most commonly included in the diet in the Blue Areas. Evidence suggests the intake of olive oil raises healthy cholesterol and reduces poor cholesterol.

In Ikaria, we find that about six tablespoons of olive oil daily appeared to decrease the chance of dying in half for middle-aged men. Whole grains and beans control the Blue Zones' diets and meals during the year, along with seasonal fruits and vegetables.

How you can do it:

- Have on deck your preferred fruits and vegetables. Seek not to push yourself to consume something you don't want. That may work a bit, but it'll flicker sooner or later. Seek a range of fruits and vegetables, learn what you want, and stock up on your fridge. Frozen vegetables are only perfect if you don't have exposure to new, healthy vegetable products. (Indeed they often produce more nutrients because they are flash-frozen at the time of harvest instead of sitting in the nearby grocery shop for weeks.)

- Use of cooking oil, for example. Olive oil seasons crops in poor sunshine. You can also use a little extra virgin olive oil on your side to finish steamed or cooked vegetables.

- Stock up grain. We found that the Blue Zones diets around the world contain peas, wheat, brown rice, and ground corn.

In those cultures, wheat was not as essential, and their grains produced less gluten than today's modern strains.

- Use some unuseful vegetables in your fridge to make vegetable soup by cutting it, browning it with olive oil and herbs and inserting boiling water to cover. Cook the vegetables until finished, then season to taste. Freeze anything you do not consume in single or family-sized containers now and only serve later in the week or month, when you do not have time for dinner.

Notes on Protein in the Blue Zones Diet

We were all advised that our bodies require protein in order to develop solid bones and muscles — but what is the right amount? The average American woman requires 70 g of protein every day, while the average American woman drinks more than 100 g of protein. It suggests from 46 to 56 grams a day in the Centers for Disease Prevention.

But quantity is not all that counts. The right type of protein is also necessary. Protein, sometimes called amino acids, are formed in 21 different varieties. Of those, the body cannot create nine; these "key" amino acids are named because we need them and need them to be derived from our diet.

All nine amino acids are supplied by meat and eggs, as well as a few herbal foods. But meat and eggs provide fat, cholesterol and cardiovascular diseases. And how are you doing when you want to follow the Blue Zones diet and show plant foods? The key is to "mix" those items. You get all the essential amino acids by mixing the right plant foods. Not only will you meet your protein requirements, but you will also control your calorie intake.

2. Retreat From Meat: Don't consume meat more than twice a week

Eat meat in quantities no greater than two ounces served twice a week or less. Enjoy real free-range chicken and family-raised pork or lamb rather than industrial-raised meats. Stop fried foods, such as hot dogs, burgers for lunch or sausages.

In most Blue Areas, diets of pork, poultry, and lamb were consumed modest quantities. Families typically slaughtered their pig or goat for summer festival festivities, eat cordially and store the leftovers which they would eventually use as fat to fry or as taste condiment. Chickens roam the ground, consume grubs and are roasted openly. However, chicken meat is also a delicacy savored over several meals.

Rationing meat intake in all of the Blue Regions, we learned that citizens consumed limited volumes of meat, two oz or less at a time, approximately five days a month. They splurged around once a month, normally on roasted pigs or goats. No beef or turkey is noticeably included in the Blue Zones regular diet.

Free-Range Meats

Meat in the blue areas is consumed by the free-roaming animals. These animals are not dosed with hormones, pesticides or antibiotics, and the misery of large feeding lots does not occur. Goats graze on grasses, leaves and herbs continually. Kitchen scraps and maize cobs and roots are consumed by Sardinian and Ikarian pigs. These conventional farming practices will yield meat with good omega-3 fatty acids higher than rich grain-fed beef.

In fact, we do not know if people would live longer if they had eaten more meat or thrived on it as part of the Blue Zones diet. There are so many safe activities in blue zones where citizens would get meat now and then since its destruction was counterbalanced by certain options of diet and lifestyles. "The better you are, the happier you become," as my buddy, Dean Ornish calls it.

How you can do it:

- Know what the two-ounce cooked meat looks like: chicken — about half chicken breast fillet or chicken leg (not skin), pork or lamb — a card deck cut, or carved into pieces, before cooking

- Stop getting steak, hot dogs, fried foods, bacon or some other product into your house because it is not included with the Blue Zones diet.

- The Americans are used to identifying food replacements for meat in a meal. Consider tofu thinly sautéed with olive oil, tempeh, another soy ingredient, or cakes of blackened bean or chickpea.

- Consume meat or other animal-derived food two days a week and just appreciate it on certain days.

- As the quantities of nearly all restaurant meat are four ounces or more, share meat with someone else or inquire in advance to carry a jar half the volume of meat back home later.

Perfect Protein Pairings

Peter J. Woolf, a chemical engineer and former University of Michigan Assistant-Professor, has collaborated with fellow scientists to define the pairings and ratios which best suit our protein needs and has studied more than 100 plant-based feed. Below are some of our dream food pairings in the Blue Zones.

Quick and Easy Snacks

- 1 1/2 cups of edamame, cooked and coated with soy sauce.

- 1⁄4 cup of walnuts plus 1 1⁄2 cups edamame, cooked.

Low-Calorie Combos from the Blue Zones Diet

- 3 cups of cooked cauliflower plus 1 1⁄3 cups chopped red peppers.
- 1 cup of cooked lentils plus 2 cups of chopped carrots.
- 1 cup of cooked chickpeas plus 3 cups of cooked mustard greens.
- 1 cup of lima beans plus 2 cups of cooked carrots.
- peas1 1⁄4 cup of cooked sweet yellow corn plus 1 cup of cooked black-eyed peas.

Extra-Filling Blue Zones Diet Dishes

- 1 cup of cooked chickpeas plus 1 1⁄4 cups of cooked brown rice
- 1 1⁄3 cup of cooked wild rice plus 1 1⁄2 cups of cooked broccoli rabe
- 1 cup of cooked brown rice plus 2⁄3 cup of extra firm tofu
- 1 1⁄4 cup of cooked soba noodles plus 1⁄2 cup of firm tofu

3. Fish Is Fine: Regularly consume up to three ounces of fish

Think about three ounces before cooking as around the size of a deck of cards. Choose local and bountiful fish that are not endangered by overfishing. The Adventist Health Study 2, which tracks 96,000 Americans since 2002, revealed that they had not become vegans or meat-eaters for the longest period. They are "Pesco-vegetarians," or fishermen, who consume a diet focused on vegetables, with a tiny portion of fish, about once a day. In other diets in the Blue Zones fish are a common part of daily meals, consumed two to three times a week on average.

Other legal and safety issues require seafood in the diet. Fish consumed in the world's blue areas are, in the majority of instances, thin, fairly cheap fish such as sardines, anchovies and cod — mid food chain organisms that are not currently subjected to high levels of mercury or other chemicals such as PCBs that pollute the source of our gourmet seafood. Humans in the blue areas are not overfishing the oceans unlike commercial fisheries, who are endangering the destruction of entire ecosystems. Fishermen in the blue areas cannot continue to wreak havoc on their reliant communities. There is no proof of the Blue Zones diet preferring other species, including salmon, however.

How you can do it:

- Know what the three ounces feel like, whether it is a larger fish's three ounces like snappers and salmon or a smaller fish's three ounces like sardines or anchovies.

- Enjoy mid-chain fish such as trunks, snappers, mixers, sardines and anchovy. Stop going for aggressive fish such as swordfish, shark or tuna to mimic a Blue Zones diet. Stop overfishing animals such as Chilean sea bass.

- Step away from "farmed" fish as typically grown in overcrowded plumes, which make antibiotics, pesticides and coloring necessary.

4. Diminish Dairy: Minimize the consumption of cow's milk and food products such as ham, sugar and butter

The Blue Zones diet includes no cow's milk noticeably, except Adventists, some of whom eat eggs and dairy items. Milk is a relative stranger to the diet of humans, added around 8,000 to 10,000 years ago. Our digestive systems are not optimized for milk or dairy (except human milk), and we now recognize that the number of people (often unwittingly) with lactose digestion difficulties can be as high as 60%.

Milk also reflects on their high content of fat and sugar. Neal Barnard, founder and chairman of the Scientific Office of Responsible Medicine, claims 49% of calories in whole foods and about 70% of calories in cheese are fat — and much of this fat is unhealthy. Both types of milk also have lactose sugar. For example, about 55% of the calories in skim milk are derived from lactose sugar.

Although Americans have relied on calcium and protein milk for decades, people in the Blue Zones diet get these nutrients from plant sources. For example, one cup of cooked kale or two-thirds of a cup of tofu provides as much organic calcium as a cup of milk.

A few days a week, a Blue Zones diet is all right with limited quantities of sheep's milk and goat's milk items – particularly full-fat, naturally fermented yoghurt without added sugar. The standard menus of the Ikarian and Sardinian Blue Zones include Goat's and sheep's dairy items prominently.

We may not know if goats' milk or sheep's milk makes people happier or if it is because humans walk up the same steep hills as the goats in the Blue Zone Areas. Interestingly, in the Blue Zone diet, the majority of goat's milk is used not as a liquid but as fermented products like yoghurt, sour milk or cheese. Although the milk of goat includes lactose, it also includes lactase, an enzyme for the digestion of lactose in the body.

How you can do it:

- Use the product as a food substitute for unsweetened corn, coconut or almond products. Most of them have the same protein as normal milk and sometimes taste decent or great.

- Fulfil the daily cheese cravings with grass-fed goats or sheep's milk. Seek the pecorino Sardo in Sardinia or the Greek feta. Both are delicious, and you just need a limited amount of food to sample.

5. Occasional Egg: Eat far more than three eggs a week

Eggs are eaten in the five Blue Zones menus, where people eat them between two to four days a week on average. Like meat protein, eggs are a side dish, eaten alongside a greater part of the whole-grain or another herbal element. To roll it the Nicoya way into a maize tortilla with a side of beans, fry an egg. For their chili, Okinawans fry an egg. The Mediterranean Blue Zones' meals are seasoned with an egg as a side dish with a breakfast of toast, almonds and olives.

Blue Zone eggs diet are obtained from widely mixed chickens that consume a vast range of natural foods, are exempted from the use of pesticides or antibiotics and yield gradually matured omega 3-acid eggs that are naturally better. Factory-producing eggs ripen half as fast as eggs laid by chickens in the Blue Areas.

Eggs have full protein with the amino acids required for your body plus B vitamins, A, D and E vitamins, and minerals such as selenium. Data from Adventist Health Study 2 revealed that vegetarians that consumed eggs live marginally longer than those who strictly eat vegetables (although they also appeared to weigh more).

There are many safety issues that may influence the choice to consume eggs in the Blue Zones diet. Diabetics must be vigilant of egg yolks, and egg intake has been associated with higher levels of men's prostate cancer and increased female kidney problems. Scholars often disagree about the impact of dietary cholesterol on lungs, but amid the specialist controversy, certain people with heart or a circulatory disorders overlook it.

How you can do it:

- Buy only cage-free, pastured chickens for small eggs.

- Complete a single egg breakfast with fruit or other natural foods, such as porridge or toast.

- Seek to swap scrambled tofu with eggs in your Blue Zone diet.

- Use a quarter of cup applesauce, a quarter cup of potatoes or a tiny banana to cover an egg when baking. Flaxseeds or agar (extracted from algae) are also used in recipes which call for eggs.

6. Daily Dose Of Beans: Eat at Least A Half Cup Normal Cooked Beans

Beans are the core of the world's Blue Zones diet: black beans in the Mediterranean; lentils, garbanzo and white beans; and soybeans in the Okinawa area. In these blue areas, the long-lived cultures consume on an average, four times as much beans as we do. A World Health Organization-funded, five-country research has shown that consuming 20 grams of beans a day lowered a person's chance of death by around 8 percent in any given year.

In reality, beans are the ideal superfood for the Blue Zones diet. On average, they contain 21% protein, 77% complex carbohydrates, and a few percent fats (this is steady and safe energy instead of the increase from processed carbohydrates including white flour). They are also a fantastic fiber supply. They are inexpensive and durable, come with a wide variety of texture and are filled with more nutrients per gram than any other Earth product.

For at least 8,000 years, humans have consumed beans; they 're part of our culinary DNA. Even Daniel's Bible Book (1:1-21) proposes a two-week bean diet for healthy babies. The typical nutritional in the Blue Areas — include at least half a cup of the vitamins and minerals you require. And since the beans are so juicy and delicious, they would presumably consume fewer nutritious foods. In fact, the high fiber content of beans lets good probiotics grow in the intestine.

How you can do it:

- Consider ways to prepare beans that tastes amazing as part of a Blue Zones diet for you and your mates. Blue Zone centenarians know how to make beans taste good. If you don't already have favorite dishes, seek three-bean dishes in the next month.

- Make sure your kitchen cupboard contains a variety of beans. Dry beans are cheapest, but boobs are faster. If you buy canned beans, make sure to read the label: beans, water, spices and maybe a little salt are the only ingredients. Avoid brands of fat or sugar added.

- Use purified beans to produce creamy, protein-rich soups on the Blue Zones diet as a thickener.

- Make salads more nutritious with grilled beans. Serve hummus or black bean cakes with additional flavor and appealing salads.

- Keep your pantry filled with condiments which serve as dressing and deliciously taste bean dishes. For starters, Mediterranean bean dishes typically include carrots, celery and onions, seasoned with garlic, thyme, pepper and bay leaves. That is an easy approach to combine a diet for the Blue Areas.

- Remember Mexican restaurants, which almost often offer pinto or black beans, as you go to eat. Add potatoes, tomatoes, mushrooms, guacamole and chili sauce to enhance the beans. Remove tortillas with white rice. Instead, pick maize tortillas to eat beans like in Costa Rica.

7. Slash Sugar: No more than seven additional teaspoons A day

Centennials typically only consume sweets only at celebrations. They do not apply sugar to their diet and usually sweeten their tea with honey. This adds up to about seven tea cubes of sugar a day in the Blue Zone diets. The lesson for us: only a few days a week, you can appreciate cakes, candy and bakeries as a dinner. Stop sugar products. Skip any substance where sugar is one of the first five specified ingredients. Limit coffee, tea or other food to a maximum of four teaspoons a day of sugar. Break the habit of snacking on fast candy with sugar.

Let's face it: Sugar can't be stopped. It exists in nuts, vegetables and milk naturally. But this isn't a problem. The sum of added sugar in food supply rose by 25 percent between 1970 and 2000. The typical person eats around 22 teaspoons of artificial sugar per day — insidious, frozen sweets found in sodas, yoghurts, muffins, and sauces. Too much sugar has been demonstrated in our diet to suppress the immune system and stop the prevention diseases. This also raises the amount of insulin that can induce diabetes and reduce productivity, render you overweight, and even shorten your life. In the Blue Zones diet, people consume around the same amount of natural sugar as North Americans, but only about one-fifth of it is from added sugars. The key: People in the Blue Zones intentionally eat sugar, not by choice or mistake.

How you can do it:

- Consider adding honey to your Blue Zones diet as sweetener. It is true that honey stimulates blood sugar much like caffeine, but it is easier to spoon in cold liquids and unlike sugar which does not melt as easily. And you would prefer to consume it more intentionally and drink less. Honey is a whole food commodity, and certain honey produces anti-inflammatory, anti-cancer and antimicrobial effects, such as Ikarian heather honey.

- Avoid sugar-sweetened sodas, teas, and fruit drinks altogether. Sugar-sweetened soda is the single biggest source of added sugars in our diet—in fact, soft drink consumption may account for 50% of America's weight gain since 1970. One can of soda pop alone contains around ten teaspoons of sugar. If you must drink sodas, choose diet soda or, better yet, seltzer or sparkling water.

- Consume sweets as a festive meal. Blue Zones people enjoy chocolate, but candies (cookies, pies, sweets of several various kinds) are almost only eaten as celebratory treats — during a Sunday dinner, during a special holiday or at a local festival. In fact, special sweets are often available for these special occasions. Restrict sweets or therapies to one hundred calories. Consume just one a day or less.

- Find fruit in the Blue Zones diet for your tasty treat. Instead of dried berries, you should consume fresh fruit. Fresh fruit have more sugar, helping you feel fuller with fewer calories. The sugars stored in dried fruits such as raisins and dates are way above what you get fresh in a traditional fresh fruit.

- Look out for packaged foods, particularly sauces, salad dressings and ketchup, with added sugar. Most produce additional sugar teaspoons.

- Look for low-fat foods, many of which are sweetened with sugar to compensate for the fat deficiency. For starters, some fatty yoghurts sometimes contain more sugar — ounce for ounce — than soda pop.

- Consider stevia to sweeten your tea or coffee if the sweet tooth doesn't end. This is definitely not a genuine aspect of the Blue Zones diet, but it is very pure and potentially healthier than processed sugar.

8. Snack On Nuts: Eat two handfuls per day of nuts

A few nuts are around two ounces, which tends to be the typical volume the centennial Blue Zones consume. In the different Blue Zones diets, nuts are consumed like almonds from Ikaria and Sardinia, pistachios from Nicoya and all the Adventist-style nuts – all nuts are fine. Nut eaters, as per the Adventist Health Study 2, outlive non-nut eaters by two or three years on average.

Similarly, a new Harvard analysis that has been tracking 100,000 people for 30 years has found that the risk of mortality in nut eaters is down by 20 percent as relative to non-nut eaters. Many tests have shown that diets of nuts decrease 'poor' LDL cholesterol by 9 to 20 per cent regardless of the amount of fat content of nuts. Copper, calcium, folate, vitamin E and arginine, an amino acid, are all good additives of nutrients.

How you can do it:

- Hold nuts for mid-morning or mid-afternoon treats in the office. Take limited transportation packages and car rides.

- Consider applying salads and soups almonds or other seeds to your meals.

- Stock a range of nuts in order to provide the food of the Blue Areas. The perfect mix: almonds (strong in vitamin E and magnesium), peanuts (high in protein and folate, vitamin B), Brazil nuts (high in selenium, a mineral thought that could defend against prostate cancer), cashews (high in magnesium), and walnuts (the only omega-three fat available are plants) are high in alpha-linolenic acid. Both these nuts will lead to raising cholesterol.

- Integrate nuts as a protein substitute into daily meals.

- To minimize total glycemic burden, consume any nuts before a meal.

9. Sour On Bread: Replace Popular Bread or 100% Whole Wheat Bread with Sourdough

For at least 10,000 years, bread has been a staple of the human diet. It remains a favorite of three of the five Blue Zones diets. While not typically used for sandwiches, it occurs at most meals. But what people in the Blue Areas consume is another bread than the bread most North Americans buy. The majority of commercially available bread begins with the white flour breed, which rapidly metabolizes in sugar. White bread contains mostly wasted calories and insulin surges. In addition, white bread (along with glucose) is the normal glycemic index score of 100 for calculating all other products.

Not only is processed sugar found in our regular white or wheat pieces of bread. Gluten, which is a grain, which gives bread its loft and shape, often makes certain people stomach issues is also found in it. The Blue Zone diet for bread is different: either whole or sourdough, each of which has its own balanced features. The bread of Icaria and Sardinia, for example, consist of wheat, rye, and barley, and both give a broad range of nutrients, for example, tryptophan, amino acid, and minerals selenium which magnesium, which comprise of 100% whole grains.

Whole grains all have higher fiber levels than wheat flours most often used. Interestingly enough, barley became the most longevity-related ingredient in Sardinia.

Many typical Blue Zones bread are produced with natural bacteria called lactobacilli, which "digest" the starches and gluten when the bread is rising. The cycle also creates an acid – the "sour" in sourdough. The effect is more gluten-free bread (about a thousandth of the gluten in regular bread), with a longer shelf life and a sweet, sour flavor, which most people prefer. Most notably, typical sourdough bread eaten in Blue Zones diets positively raises the glycemic load of food. It helps make the whole meal safer, quicker to cook, better on the pancreas and more likely to contain calories as energy than fat.

Be mindful that industrial sourdough in products may differ significantly and therefore does not have the same nutritional characteristics as conventional natural sourdough. Shop from a revered — presumably nearby — bakery and ask their starts if you want to purchase organic sourdough bread. A bakery which can not address the query presumably doesn't produce true sourdough bread, which should not be used in your Blue Zones diet.

How you can do it:

- If you consume bread, make sure it's real sourdough bread, like they do in Ikaria. This slow-rising bread is produced with lactobacteria, also referred to as pain au levain, as an agent that does not contain industrial yeast.

- Consider getting yourself sourdough bread from a real sourdough starter. Ed Wood, a regional geographical writer buddy, provides some of the finest details on sourdough and on sourdo.com stats.

- Seek the Blue Zones diet of brown grain pasta. Experts claim that as grains are sprouting, starches and proteins become harder to absorb. Proven bread often gives higher levels of functional iron, than regular grain types, and important amino acids, minerals and B vitamins. Ounce for ounce, sprouts are known to be one of the most healthy foods.

- Pick wholegrain rye or pumpernickel bread for whole wheat: the glycemic index is smaller. See the label, however. Avoid rye bread which lists wheat flour as their first ingredient and look for the first ingredient of the bread that lists rye flour. Most breads in the store are not real bread of rye.

- Select or make bread that contains seeds, nuts, dried fruits and whole grains. A whole food such as flaxseed provides flavor, variety, density and nutritional value.

- Check for (or bake) fresh barley bread with 75% to 80% whole-barley kernels on average.

- In general, it is the sort you can recognize if you can fit a slice of the bread into a sphere. Look for hard, packed 100% whole-grain bread, which is minimally refined.

10. Go Wholly Whole: Eat meals and what you will remember

Another concept of 'real food' would be a single product, fresh, fried, roasted or fermented, and not strongly prepared. (For example, Tofu is not very much processed whereas cheese doodles and frozen sausage dogs are highly processed.) Historically, people are eating the whole food across the Blue Zones and in their diets worldwide. They do not throw away the yolk to produce an egg-blank omelet or to spin the fat out of the yoghurt or to juice apple from the fruit to the fiber-rich pulp. They do not intensify or add additional ingredients to change their foods' nutritional profile. They get all they need from nutrient-dense fiber-rich foods instead of vitamins or other nutrients. And when cooking meals, such dishes usually contain half a dozen or so of ingredients, which are easily combined together.

Nearly all the food consumed for hundreds of years in the Blue Zones – up to 90% – are also produced in a ten-mile radius. Preparation of food is quick. You eat crude fruits and vegetables, you grind whole grains and slowly cook them. Fermentation is an ancient way of availing nutrients in tofu, sourdough, wine and spices they consume.

Only consume natural foods, and residents in the blue areas rarely eat chemicalized food. The foods they eat are digested slowly, particularly grains, so blood sugar does not spike. Nutrition biologists are only just beginning to understand how all elements of the whole plants (rather than individual nutrients) function synergistically together to maintain optimal wellbeing. Several thousands of phytonutrients – naturally occurring plant nutrients – are still to be identified.

How you can do it:

- Shop in farmer markets or on town-sponsored farms. Avoid foods wrapped in plastic.
- Avoid factory-made foods.
- Stop more than five food nutritional component items.
- Avoid pre-made or ready-to-eat meals.
- At least three Super Blue Zone Foods a day should be consumed. You don't have to consume these things in bulk. Yet you'll also find that these ingredients go on to improve your stamina and strength and that you're less inclined to switch to the sugar and unhealthy, fried stuff that offers you the "fix" instantly (and quickly goes away).

11. Eat Super Blue Zone Foods: Integrate into your routine the blue zones diet to ensure sure that you consume plenty of whole food

- **Beans**—all kinds: pinto beans, black beans, garbanzo beans, lentils, black-eyed peas
- **Greens**— beet tops, spinach, kale, chards, fennel tops
- **Sweet potatoes**—don't confuse with yams
- **Nuts**—all kinds: Brazil nuts, almonds, walnuts, peanuts, sunflower seeds, cashews
- **Olive oil**—green, Typically, extra-virgin is the highest. (Note that olive oil decomposes rapidly, so purchase a supply at a period of no more than one month.)
- **Oats**—slow-cooking or Irish steel-cut are best
- **Barley**— in soups, as soft rice, or bread flour
- **Fruits**—all kinds
- **Green or herbal teas**
- **Turmeric**—as a spice or a tea

12. The Blue Zones Beverage Rules: Drink Coffee For Bed, Tea In The Afternoon, Champagne At 5:00 P.M. Never drink soda water, including diet soda

People in Blue Zones drink beer, coffee, tea and wine with a few exceptions. (The bulk of Blue Zone Centenarians do not recognize Soda Pop, which accounts for around half America's sugar consumption.) There is a clear reason behind that.

Health: Seven glasses of health are expressly prescribed every day by Adventists. Research suggests that being amply hydrated allows for blood supply to be smoother and lessens the risk of blood coagulation. I assume that there is one extra benefit: if people consume water, then they will not consume a drink full of sugar (soda, fuel drinks and fruit juices) or a chemically sweetened product, both of which may be carcinogenic.

Coffee: Sardinians, Icarian and Nicoya's all have plenty of coffee. Research studies link coffee consumption to lower obesity levels and Parkinson's disease. However, coffee appears to be a shade-grown in the blue areas of the planet, an activity that favors birds and the climate, another illustration of how diets in blue areas represent a broader picture.

Tea: Tea is drunk by men in the Blue Zones. Okinawan's nursing green tea has been shown to reduce the risks of cardiac disease and a number of cancers generally. Icarians drink rosemary, wild sage and dandelion brews — all of which are known to have anti-inflammatory characteristics.

Red Wine: People who drink tend to survive longer than those who don't. Residents in most Blue Zones consume one or three bottles of wine a day, sometimes with dinners and mates. (This does not mean you can consume because you don't drink right now.) In addition, wine has been shown to help the body digest plant-based antioxidants and complements a Blue Zone diet in particular. Such advantages may come from resveratrol, a red wine-specific antioxidant. Yet, a little alcohol may also help lift depression at the end of the day, which is beneficial for mental wellbeing. In either event, women and men have negative health consequences over two or three glasses a day. For women, less than one drink a day raises the risk of breast cancer.

How you can do it:

- Keep a full bottle of water in your desk or workplace and by the bed.

- Have a cup of coffee to begin the day. Coffee is mildly sweetened and drank plain without milk in blue zones diets.

- Stop coffee after midnight as caffeine will conflict with sleep (and, by the way, hundreds of years old get an average of 8 hours a night).

- Be free to drink green tea all day long. Green tea typically produces about 25% more caffeine than coffee and delivers a steady supply of antioxidants.

- Seek various herbal teas including rosemary, oregano or sage.

- Sweeten the teas with sweet honey gently and hold them in the fridge reservoir for easy access in hot weather.

- Never bring soda pop into your house.

Developing A Taste for Blue Zones Foods

If I've done my job so far, I've entertained you with suggestions on approaches you can use to improve your own food options like people in the Blue Zone Areas. I have provided you with a selection of foodstuffs that the longest-lived people in the world consume, along with guidance on their preference, preparation and feeding. But what if you and your family don't like the food on that list, even though it is part of the Blue Zones diet? I could tell you that broccoli and beans are good for you all day long. So you might consume broccoli and beans for some time, so ultimately you'll tire of them and go back to consuming what you're used to.

Fear of sugar and resistance to bitterness is something almost everybody is born with. That is because sugar, in fact, implies calories and also bitterness indicates pollutants. Early humans who gravitated to sweets and berries were more likely nibbling bitter-tasting plants to thrive, including greens which supply vitamins, minerals, and fiber that today are a prominent feature of Blue Zones diets. We would obviously favor chocolate bars over broccoli or sprouts in Brussels.

We are all born with the tastes of our mothers for a certain cuisine. We are likely to be born with a preference for junk food because our mothers eat salty foods rich in saturated and Trans-fats during their pregnancy. Alternatively, if a mother eats a lot of garlic before conception, the amniotic fluid will feel like garlic, and the infant will probably taste it. If your mother wasn't a healthy eater, as many women, who were got pregnant after 1950, you undoubtedly were raised with disabilities.

Finally, most of our tastes are formed at the age of five. Indeed, the best time to acquire new flavors is the first year of life. Sadly, most new mothers do not know and feed their children porridge or sweetened baby foods, which tend the taste of the children to live on junk foods. Or give in to the ease of buying salty, fat snacks for their babies. In Blue Areas, mothers feed their kids with several of the same whole products, such as rice, whole-grain porridges and mashed-up berries. (French fries are the most widely eaten by 15-month old kids in the United States).

So what are the easiest approaches to bring yourself and your families to the right nutritional choices? To find out, I called Leann L. Birch of Penn State Department of Nutrition and Marcia Pelchat of Philadelphia's Monell Chemical Senses Center, who are flavor experts. I found that we don't only learn to like new foods throughout our lives, but that there's a scientific approach to learning how to like food that is good for you. They showed me the fundamentals to help kids enjoy fresh nutritious foods like vegetables. Such methods can often work with adults with minor changes.

How you can do it for kids:

- Children are usually cautious about new foods, so make new vegetables that are common to be enticing to your kid. When used to pure milk, start out offering new soft or heavy vegetables when cooked. If your child loves crispy, crunchy food, then raw veggies are presented.

- Before a meal or as a first course introduce fresh food if children are hungry.

- Do not force foods on kids. You can turn them off for life.

- Introduce a range of Blue Zone diet items. Your children can be instinctively attracted to peas and carrots, but they can dislike broccoli and green beans. Serve little of a half dozen vegetables at a time, a kind of Blue Zone's succotash, and see what the children want best. If you learn that, you should continue to plan these latest favorites in different ways.

How you can do it for adults:

- Discover what you like. Take a peek at the above notes about how children develop tastes and try different foods, for example, before eating, if you are tired.

- Learn some new cooking skills. You should not consume vegetables unless you learn how to make them in an appealing way.

- Take a vegetarian cooking class.

- Host a Blue Zones potluck. Share the Blue Zones diet with your mates and food guidelines and the compilation of ten Special Blue Zone Items. Request all to bring a plate with one or two of these items. Every one of you can use your culinary skills to try new plant-based foods and improve your social network — one of the main objectives of those who want to raise life like in the Blue Zones.

13. Four Always, Four to Avoid

It took my team a long time to establish the above 10 Blue Zones food and diet guidelines. Which may be far too dramatic for certain people to alter the food they have consumed for most of their lives.

Brian Wansink of Cornell, Leslie Lytle University of Minnesota and a couple of others worked together to discuss the best and worst recipes for them. We also set down certain criteria:

• Foods must "Always" be easily available and inexpensive.

• "Always" food must taste fine and be reasonably flexible to use in most meals.

• Items "to avoid" should be closely associated with hypertension, heart failure or cancer and excessive tension in the regular diet in the United States.

• Both food terms "always" and "To Stop" needed to be backed up with solid facts.

Here's what we came up with and what any choice is behind.

Four Always

It may be better to identify four food classes than recalling all the items that have been cooked in the Blue Zones diet.

The following include:

1. 100% Whole Wheat Bread: We figured it could be toasted in the morning and rendered a balanced lunch sandwich. While maybe not the ideal longevity meal, it may help eliminate white bread from the

diet and represent a significant step in most Americans' direction towards a balanced blue zone diet.

2. Nuts: We realize the nut eaters endure those who eat noodles. Nuts come in a wide varieties and are packed with nutrients and healthy fat to feed the appetite. The perfect snack is a two-ounce mix of nuts (a few of them). You will preferably hang on to tiny two-ounce packets. Small amounts are better as oils decay (oxidize) in nuts. Larger volumes can be kept for a couple of months in the refrigerator or freezer.

3. Beans: I claim that beans of all sorts are the main longevity commodity of the world. They are simple, flexible and filled with nutrients, vitamins and fiber that are delightful to taste. It is safer to purchase dried beans and to cook them quickly, but low-sodium canned beans in non-BPA cans are all right. Know how to cook with beans and store them dry, and you'll make a major jump to a Blue Zones diet.

4. Your Favorite Fruit: Buy a lovely bowl of fruit, place it in the middle of your kitchen (on the wall, the central island or the table,

anywhere you go the most), and place it under the sun. Data indicates that we really consume what we see, and that's what we're going to eat if we just have chips in the door. But if you want a fruit and keep it in plain view all the way, you are likely to consume some of it and feel happier with it. Don't hesitate to buy fruit you know you can consume, unless you just don't want it.

Four to Avoid

Similarly, recalling four laws about what foods will support Blue Zone, and those that deter from it, not being in your fridge and kitchen cupboard as it might make the cycle simpler. We don't mean you should never treat yourself with such products. Indeed, if you enjoy all of these products and you are happy, you can sometimes indulge completely. But reserve them for celebration or, at least, making sure you bring them down. Don't put them in your home and then with so much sadness, you'll end up removing all of the harmful items that don't occur in the Blue Zone diet.

1. Sugar-Sweetened Beverages: Harvard's Willett reported that 50% of the caloric intake in America was primarily due to empty calories and liquefied sugar in sodas and bottled juices. Will you ever place your cereal with ten teaspoons of sugar? Probably not. However,

that's how much sugar you drink when you get a 12-unce soda pop bowl.

2. Salty Snacks: We invest approximately 6 billion dollars a year on potato chips — a food (maybe not by chance) often correlated with obesity (although fast-closing pork rinds). Nearly all chips and crackers contain large concentrations of salt, preservatives and heavily refined grains, metabolizing rapidly into sugar. They were also specially designed to be crunchy and delicious and to offer a sultry mouth feeling. They are built to be irresistible, in other words. And how are you stopping them? Don't let them school you!

3. Processed Meats: More than half a million individuals have observed a new epidemiology report over the past decades, which has shown that those who consume significant quantities of sausages, salami, burgers, lunch meats and other heavily prepared foods had the highest levels of cancer and heart disease. Again, the threat here is double. These meat products have been known to have carcinogenic substances such as nitrates and other preservatives. They are doing their job and preserving the products well, meaning that processed meats are readily in the store at home or in the shop,

for snacking or quick meals, which is not same for households and diets in the Blue Zones.

4. Packaged Sweets: Including crispy chips, biscuits, cakes, muffins, granola bars and even nutrition bars, all of them produce a variety of spicy insulin fat. We are all genetically vivacious in our hunt for candy, and we want naturally to fulfil an urge by opening and digging in a box of cookies. Blues Zone diet classes will advise us that if you decide to make cookies or a cake and get it all round, all right. When you like the odd delicious goodness in your corner shop, fine, but just don't stack your cupboard of packed sucrose treats.

I have put together all longevity foods into a single page, below, for your convenience. Pick as many as possible, know how to train them, stay with them for a long time, and see how good they are.

14. Longevity Superfoods from the World's Blue Zones Diets:

Vegetables

- Wakame (seaweed)
- Fennel

- Kombu (seaweed)

- Shiitake mushrooms

- Potatoes

- Sweet potatoes

- Wild greens

- Squash

- Yams

Fruits

- Avocados

- Tomatoes

- Bananas

- Bitter melons

- Papayas

- Lemons

- Plantains

- Pejivalles (peach palms)

Beans (Legumes)

- Chickpeas

- Black beans

- Black-eyed peas
- Other cooked beans
- Fava beans

Grains

- Brown rice
- Barley
- Whole-grain bread
- Oatmeal
- Maize nixtamal

Nuts and Seeds

- Other nuts
- Almonds

Lean Protein

- Soy milk
- Salmon
- Tofu

Dairy

- Pecorino cheese
- Feta cheese

Added Oils

- Olive oil

Beverages

- Red wine
- Coffee
- Water
- Green tea

Sweeteners and Seasonings

- Garlic
- Mediterranean herbs
- Honey
- Turmeric

- Milk thistle

SIRTFOOD RECIPES

1. SIRTFOOD BITES

Ingredients:

- (85% cocoa solids), 1 ounce (30g) of dark chocolate, 1/4 cup of cocoa nibs or broken into pieces
- 1 cup (120g) of walnuts
- , 9 ounces (250g) of pitted Medjool dates
- One tablespoon of ground turmeric
- One tablespoon of cocoa powder
- The scraped seeds of 1 vanilla pod or one teaspoon of vanilla extract
- One tablespoon of extra virgin olive oil
- 1 to 2 tablespoons of water

Instructions:

- Place the walnuts and the chocolate in a food processor and then Proceed until you've got a fine powder.
- Add all other ingredients other than water and combine until a ball is shaped. Depending on the consistency of the mixture, you may or may not add the water — you don't want it to be too gummy.

- Make a bite-sized paste with your hands and cool them down for at least 1 hour in an airtight jar before consuming them.
- You can roll some of the balls to a different finish if you want to, in some cocoa or dried cocoa. You can leave in your fridge for up to 1 week.

2. *SIRT SUPER SALAD*

Ingredients:

- 1 3⁄4 ounces (50g) of endive leaves
- 1 3⁄4 ounces (50g) of arugula
- 3 1⁄2 ounces (100g) of smoked salmon slices
- 1⁄2 cup (50g) of celery including leaves, sliced
- 1⁄2 cup (80g) of avocado, peeled, stoned, and sliced
- 1⁄8 cups (15g) of walnuts, chopped
- 1⁄8 cup (20g) of red onion, sliced
- One tablespoon of capers
- One tablespoon of extra virgin olive oil
- One large Medjool date, pitted and chopped
- Juice of 1⁄4 lemon
- 1⁄4 cup (10g) of parsley, chopped

Instructions:

- In a plate or wide cup, place the salad leaves.

- Mix all the remaining ingredients and pour over the seeds.

3. MISO-MARINATED BAKED COD WITH STIR-FRIED GREENS AND SESAME

Ingredients:

- One tablespoon of extra virgin olive oil
- 3 1/2 teaspoons (20g) of miso
- One tablespoon of mirin
- 1/8 cup (20g) of a red onion, sliced
- 1 x 7-ounce (200g) of skinless cod fillet
- Two garlic cloves, finely chopped
- 3/8 cup (40g) of celery, sliced
- One teaspoon of finely chopped fresh ginger
- One Thai chili, finely chopped
- 3/4 cup (50g) of kale, roughly chopped
- 3/8 cup (60g) of green beans
- Two tablespoons (5g) of parsley, roughly chopped
- One teaspoon of sesame seeds
- 1/4 cup (40g) of buckwheat
- One tablespoon of tamari (or soy sauce, if not avoiding gluten)
- One teaspoon of ground turmeric

Instructions:

- Combine the miso, mirin and one teaspoon of olive oil. Rub the mix all over the whole cod and set for 30 minutes to marinate. Oven heated to 220 degrees C (425 degrees F).

- Bake the cod for 10 minutes.

- Heat up the remaining oil in a large frying pan or wok. Add the celery, garlic, chili, ginger, green beans, and kale and fry for a few minutes. Turn until the kale is soft and cooked. To help the cooking process, you might have to put a bit of water into the pot.

- Cook buckwheat together with turmeric in accordance with the package instructions.

- Serve the stir-fry with sesame, parsley, tamari seeds and fish. Serve in the stir-fry.

4. AROMATIC CHICKEN BREAST WITH KALE AND RED ONIONS AND A TOMATO AND CHILI SALSA

Ingredients:

- Skinless 1/4 pound (120 g), Monotonous chicken breast.

- Two ground turmeric teaspoons

- 1/2 a lemon's juice

- One tablespoon of extra virgin olive oil.

- Three-quarters (50 g) kale, chopped.

- Red onion, chopped - 1/8 cup (20 g)

- One teaspoon of Fresh ginger, sliced

- 1/3 cup of light wheat (50 g)

The Salsa

- One small (130 g) tomato

- One Thai chili, thinly sliced.

- One teaspoon of caper, fine cut

- Parsley - 2 teaspoons (5 g), fine cut

- 1/4 of a lemon's juice

Instructions:

- Remove the eye from the tomato to make the salsa and slice it finely, ensuring that the fluid remains in as much as possible. Combine chile, capers, lemon juice and parsley. You might mix it all in, but the end product is a little different.

- Oven to 220 degrees Celsius (425 ° F), in one teaspoon, marinate the chicken breast with a little oil and lemon juice. Leave for five to ten minutes.

- Then add the marinated chicken and cook on either side for about a minute, until pale golden, transfer to the oven (on a baking tray, if your pan is not ovenproof), 8 to 10 minutes or until cooked. Remove from the oven, cover with tape, and wait until eaten for five minutes.

- Cook the kale for 5 minutes in a steamer in the meantime, add a little butter, fry the red onions and the ginger and then mix in the fluffy but not browned mix.

- Cook the buckwheat with the remaining teaspoon of turmeric according to the package instructions. Eat rice, tomatoes and salsa. Eat together.

5. ASIAN SHRIMP STIR-FRY WITH BUCKWHEAT NOODLES

Ingredients:

- Two teaspoons of tamari (you can use soy sauce if you are not avoiding gluten)
- 1/3 pound (150g) of shelled raw jumbo shrimp, deveined
- Two teaspoons of extra virgin olive oil
- Two garlic cloves, finely chopped
- Three ounces (75g) of soba (buckwheat noodles)
- One teaspoon of finely chopped fresh ginger
- One Thai chili, finely chopped
- 1/2 cup (45g) of celery including leaves, trimmed and sliced, with leaves set aside
- 1/8 cup (20g) of red onions, sliced
- 3/4 cup (50g) of kale, roughly chopped
- 1/2 cup (75g) of green beans, chopped
- 1/2 cup (100ml) of chicken stock

Instructions:

- Prepare the pan on high heat, then cook the shrimps for 2 to 3 minutes with 1 tamari teaspoon and one olive oil teaspoon.

- Switch to a tray of shrimp. Cover the pan with a towel or cloth, and you'll need it again.

- Cook the noodles for 5 to 8 minutes or as indicated on the box in boiling water. Drain and reserve.

- Fry the garlic, pepper, ginger and red onion, celery (but not the blade) over half to high heat for 2 to 3 minutes in the remaining tamari and oil. Stir in the stock and boil until they are tender, but crunchy, then simmer for a minute or two.

- Stir in a pan and put back to boil, then take the shrimp, pasta, and celery leaves from the oven, and eat.

6. ASIAN SHRIMP STIR-FRY WITH BUCKWHEAT NOODLES

Ingredients:

- Two teaspoons of tamari (you can use soy sauce if you are not avoiding gluten).
- 1/3 pound (150g) of shelled raw jumbo shrimp, deveined.
- Two teaspoons of extra virgin olive oil
- Two garlic cloves, finely chopped
- 3 ounces (75g) of soba (buckwheat noodles)
- One teaspoon of finely chopped fresh ginger
- 1 Thai chili, finely chopped
- 1/2 cup (45g) of celery including leaves, trimmed and sliced, with leaves set aside
- 1/8 cup (20g) of red onions, sliced
- 3/4 cup (50g) of kale, roughly chopped
- 1/2 cup (75g) of green beans, chopped
- 1/2 cup (100ml) of chicken stock

Instructions:

- Cover the pot over high heat and cook the shrimp for 2-3 minutes in 1 teaspoon of tamari and one teaspoon of butter.

- Move the shrimp a plate. Remove the saucepan with a cloth, as you will use the towel again.

- Cook the noodles for 5 to 8 minutes or as indicated on the package in boiling water, drain and reserve.

- In the meantime, put the sauce on medium to high heat for 2 to 3 minutes, fry the garlic, chili, ginger, red onion, celery (not the leaves), green beans and add in the remaining tamari and oil. Add the stock and leave to boil then simmer until the vegetables are crunchy and cooked, for a minute or two.

- Add the pan with shrimp, noodles and celery leaves, bring back to boil and serve off the heat.

7. STRAWBERRY BUCKWHEAT TABBOULEH

Ingredients:

- One tablespoon of ground turmeric
- 1/3 cup (50g) of buckwheat
- 1/2 cup (80g) of avocado
- 1/8 cup (20g) of red onion
- 3/8 cup (65g) of tomato

- One tablespoon of capers
- 1/8 cup (25g) of Medjool dates, pitted
- 2/3 cup (100g) of strawberries, hulled
- 3/4 cup (30g) of parsley
- Juice of 1/2 a lemon
- One tablespoon of extra virgin olive oil
- 1 ounce (30g) of arugula

Instructions:

- Cook the buckwheat with the turmeric according to the directions on the box.
- Rinse and drain to cool off.
- Chop the tomato finely, peppers, red onions, dates, capers, and pots, and mix along with the fresh buckwheat.
- Dice the strawberries and combine the oils with the lemon juice softly in the salad. Serve on arugula bed.

8. SIRTFOOD GREEN JUICE

Ingredients:

- A large handful (1 ounce or 30g) of arugula
- Two large handfuls (about 2 1/2 ounces or 75g) of kale

- 2 to 3 large celery stalks (5 1⁄2 ounces or 150g), including leaves

- A very small handful (about 1⁄4 ounce or 5g) of flat-leaf parsley

- 1⁄2 to 1-inch (1 to 2.5 cm) piece of fresh ginger

- 1⁄2 of a medium sized green apple

- 1⁄2 teaspoon of matcha powder

- juice of 1⁄2 a lemon

Instructions:

- Mix the greens together and then sauté the greens. We discovered that the efficiency of juicers could vary greatly from leafy food to rejuvenate the rest of the food, before moving to other ingredients. The goal is to get approximately 2 or 1⁄4 cup of green juice or around two fluid ounces.

- Add Celery juice, apple juice, ginger juice

- You can peel and place the citrus fruit also, but it is much easier to just squeeze the citrus fruits by hand into the juice. By this point, you should have a limit of about 1 cup (250 ml) of water.

- You just add the matcha if the juice is made and ready to drink. Into a glass, add a small amount of the juice and mix with a blaze or teaspoon vigorously.

- Add the rest of the juice when the matcha is dissolved. Give it a quick swirl, and then drink. Feel free to enhance the palate with plain water.

9. SIRT MUESLI (SERVES 1)

To make it in bulk or to make it overnight, simply put the dry ingredients together and store it in a container. Only apply the strawberries and yoghurt the next day, and it's ready to go.

Ingredients:

- 10g buckwheat puffs
- 20g buckwheat flakes
- 100g strawberries, hulled and chopped
- 15g coconut flakes or desiccated coconut
- 15g walnuts, chopped
- 40g Medjool dates, pitted and chopped
- 10g cocoa nibs

- 100g plain Greek yoghurt (or vegan alternative, such as soya or coconut yoghurt)

Instructions:

- Mix all of these products together (leave the fruits and yoghurt out if you aren't instantly serving).

10. MATCHA WITH VANILLA

Prep: 5 Mins, Easy Serves: 1

Swap the tasty green matcha and the white tea in this Japanese-style tea or coffee. It's easy to make at home, and it only takes 5 minutes.

Ingredients:

- Seeds from half a vanilla pod
- ½ tsp of matcha powder

Instruction:

- Heat the kettle then apply 100ml of water to it. In a tiny cup, pour half the hot water, steam and then transfer the matcha powder and vanilla seeds to the remaining water in the cup.

- Stir the mixture up to a smooth, slightly smooth and lump-free matcha with a bamboo whisk or mini-electric whisk. In the hot teapot, remove the water and then dump the cooked matcha tea into it.

11. TURMERIC TEA

Prep: 5 Mins, Cook: 5 Mins, Easy   Serves 2

Go to the spice rack and take turmeric to create this coffee-free drink. This orange spice occurs everywhere on the menus.

Ingredients:

- 1 tbsp of fresh grated ginger
- 3 heaped tsp of ground turmeric
- honey or agave and lemon slices, to serve
- One small orange, zest pared

Instructions:

- Boil water in a 500ml tea pot. In another teapot or jug, put turmeric, ginger and orange zest. Sprinkle with the hot water for about 5 minutes.
- Strain into two cups using a sieve or Tea strainer, apply a slice of lemon and sweeten, whether you prefer, with sweet honey or agave.

12. Date And Walnut Cinnamon Bites

PREP: 5 MINS, No Cook, EASY   SERVES 1

These cinnamon dates and walnut bites are quick to whip up for a good snack. They act even as a reward when you have friends.

Ingredients:

- Three pitted Medjool dates
- Three walnut halves
- Add the ground cinnamon, to taste

Instruction:

- Split each walnut half carefully into three pieces and then do the same with the dates. Place on top of every date a piece of walnut and cover with cinnamon dust.

13. RED CHICORY, PEAR AND HAZELNUT SALAD

Ingredients:

For the dressing:

- 1 tsp of sherry or cider vinegar
- Two heads of red chicory or white if not available
- 25g of hazelnuts, toasted and chopped

- Two ripe red Williams pears

- A good handful of rocket leaves

- 2 tbsp of hazelnut or olive oil

- 1 tsp of green peppercorns in brine, optional

- 2 tbsp. of salad oil, either sunflower oil or safflower oil.

Instructions:

- Dress up. If using green peppercorn, lightly crush them in a bowl or use a pestle and mortar with a wooden spoon. Mix the oils and vinegar and sprinkle with the salt.

- Remove the stalk from the chicory and any tired looking external leaves. Break the leaves carefully and organize in 4 sections-whether each one is big, cut or torn.

- Take the tongs out of the pears, and lengthwise quarter the pears. Cut the kernel and dice the fruit thinly. Arrange the chicory slices and spoon more than half of the sauce. Pour the remaining dressing, salt and pepper seasoning over the rocket leaves. Place the leaves on top of each salad and easily flip. Sprinkle and top with almonds.

14. *ITALIAN KALE*

Prep: 5 Mins, Cook: 5 Mins, Easy   Serves 8

This vibrant green lateral dish was tasted and dressed in vinegar, giving it a sweet and sour taste which keeps you coming back for more.

Ingredients:

- Three tbsp of red wine vinegar
- Three garlic cloves, finely sliced
- Three tbsp of olive oil
- 300g cavolo nero or kale, roughly shredded

Instructions:

- Then apply the vinegar and a splash of water to heat the oil into a large bowl with a plate, fill it with the garlic.
- Top up the kale and cover the steam, adding more water if the pot gets too dry for 4-5 minutes. Season with a little sea salt once the kale gets wilted.

15. BROCCOLI AND KALE GREEN SOUP

Prep: 15 Mins, Cook: 20 Mins, Easy Serves 2

This super healthy soup combines broccoli with ginger, coriander and turmeric to make a dense and fat lunch with nutrients.

Ingredients:

- One tbsp of sunflower oil
- 500ml, by mixing powder of 1 tbsp broth and boiling water in a jug
- Two garlic cloves, sliced
- Sliced ½ tsp of ground coriander, thumb-sized piece ginger.
- 1/2 tsp of fresh turmeric root, peeled and grated.
- 85g broccoli
- 100g kale, chopped
- 200g courgettes, roughly sliced
- One lime, zested and juiced
- A thin, finely chopped parsley pack with a few whole leaves.

Instructions

- In a deep pot, place the butter, add the garlic, ginger, coriander, salt and turmeric, and fry over medium heat for 2 minutes, then add 3 tbsp of water, give the spices a little more moisture.

- Add the courgettes, ensure that the slices have a good mixture of all the spices, then cook 3 minutes. Add stock of 400 ml and cook for 3 minutes.

- Add the remaining stock to the broccoli, kale and lime juice. Let all vegetables soften and cook once more for 3-4 minutes.

- Turn off the heat and add the pickled parsley. Load it all into a machine and blend it easily to high speed. It'll be a pretty leaf with patches of shadow (the kale). Decorate with parsley and lime.

16. STRAWBERRY, TOMATO AND POTATO SALAD WITH HONEY & PINK PEPPER DRESSING

Prep: 10 Mins, Cook: 2 Mins, Easy Serves 4

As a side meal, or even for lunch on your own, eat this cherry, tomato and potato salad. Pink peppers offer a gentle spice in the dressing

Ingredients:

- 100g potatoes
- 300g strawberries
- Three tbsp of extra virgin olive oil

- Two strawberries (about 40g), chopped

For the dressing:

- Three tbsp of pink peppercorns
- ½ lemon, juiced
- ½ tbsp of honey
- 250g mixed tomatoes

Instructions:

- Toast the potatoes with a dry pot for 1-2 minutes, then cook quickly with a stick and a touch of Salt to split up the skins.
- To prepare the sauce. Attach and crush the two strawberries into a paste.

- Stir in the lemon juice and the honey. In a large bowl, put the dressing and the olive oil whisk. Please check the seasoning and if you like add a bit more salt or lemon juice. To assemble the bowl, split the strawberries into quarters or thin wedges, and finely slice the tomatoes, chopping some and halving others, so you get plenty of various shapes. In the bowl, mix with the hammer.

- Place the salad on a tray to serve

17. ORIENTAL SALMON AND BROCCOLI TRAYBAKE

Prep: 10 Mins, Cook: 20 Mins, Easy Serves 4

Everything you need to create this Asian flavored fish dish with balanced greens and fresh lemon is five ingredients.

Ingredients:

- One head of broccoli, broken into florets
- Four skin-on salmon fillets
- juice ½ lemon, ½ lemon quartered
- Two tbsp of soy sauce
- small bunch spring onions, sliced

Instructions:

- 180C/160C heating stove/gas
- Place the salmon in a large tin to roast, making space for each fillet.

- Wash and dry broccoli and arrange around the fillets, while still a little wet. Sprinkle the lemon juice on top, then apply the quarter of a lemon.

- Sprinkle half the onions with a little olive oil on top and add them to the oven for 14 minutes. Remove from the oven, sprinkle it with the soy, return to the oven for another 4 minutes before salmon is ready. Just before serving, sprinkle with the remaining spring onions.

18. SUPERHEALTHY SALMON SALAD

PREP: 20 MINS, COOK: 5 MINS, Ready In 25 Minutes, EASY

SERVES: 2

Super-healthy by word, super-healthy by nature: This salad is rich in omega-3, iron and calcium and counts as 2 of your five a day salad.

Ingredients:

- Two salmon fillets
- 100g couscous
- 1 tbsp olive oil
- juice one lemon
- 200g sprouting broccoli, roughly shredded, larger stalks removed
- a small handful of pumpkin seeds
- seeds from half a pomegranate
- Two handfuls of watercress
- olive oil and extra lemon wedges, to serve

Instruction:

- Heat a stage steamer with gas. Season the couscous, then sprinkle with 1 tsp oil. Pour water over the couscous and cover it by 1 cm, then set aside. When the water in the steamer begins to simmer, tip the broccoli into the water and then place the salmon in the above stage—Cook for 3 minutes before the salmon is finished, and broccoli is tender. Drain the broccoli and refrigerate under the cool spray.

- Add the remaining oil and lemon juice together. Toss the broccoli, pomegranate seeds and the pumpkin seeds with the lemon dressing through the couscous. Chop the watercress loosely at the last minute, then throw into the couscous. Serve, if you want, with the tuna, lemon wedges to squeeze over it and fresh olive oil to drizzle.

19. MALABAR PRAWNS

Prep: 15 Mins, Cook: 12 Mins, Easy Serves 4

Create one a favorite dish, Kerala-Malabar prawns, a South Indian coast specialty. They are fast and easy to prepare and filled with distinct flavors

Ingredients:

- 400 grams of frozen king prawns
- 2 tsp turmeric
- Kashmiri chili powder, 3-4 tsp.
- 4 tsp of Lemon juice, with pinch
- 40gm ginger, half peeled and dried, half finely cut in similar lines.

- Vegetable oil, 1 tbsp.

- Four Leaves of curry.

- Two - Four oranges

- Halves of healthy chilies

- One fine-sliced onion.

- One tsp of black pepper cracked.

- 40gm new rubbed coconut.

- 1/2 batch of coriander, leaves only

Instructions:

- Wash the prawns in cold water, then dry pick. Toss them and put aside with the turmeric, chili powder, lemon juice, and ginger in a mix.

- Heat the oil in a saucepan and add the curry leaves, chili, sliced ginger and onion. Cook for around 10 mins until translucent, then apply the black pepper.

- Stir-fry the prawns with some marinade once tender, around 2 minutes. Season and apply a squeeze of lemon juice if necessary. Serve with coconut and leaves of coriander added.

20. CHICKEN, KALE AND SPROUT STIR-FRY

Prep: 10 Mins, Cook: 20 Mins, Easy Serves: 2

Brussels sprouts are not enough for Christmas - add them for extra protein and crunch in a balanced noodle dish.

Ingredients:

- 100 g noodle soba.
- 100 g curly shredded broccoli.
- Sesame Oil, 2 tsp.
- Two lean breasts of meat, skin off, cut into thin pieces.
- 25 g fresh ginger, peeled and cut into matching rods.
- One hot, required, thin-sliced pepper
- Handful sprouting of Brussels, sliced into pieces.
- One tbsp of soy sauce, low sodium
- 2 tbsp rice wine or vinegar with white wine
- One lime juice and zest.

Instructions:

- Cook the noodles according to the directions for packaging, then drain and set aside. In the meantime, heat a large wok or frying pan and add the kale with a good splash of water and cook for 1-2 minutes, but leave with a remaining crunch, then cool under running water to keep the color.

- Add half of the oil and cook the strips of chicken until browned, then cut and put aside. Heat the remaining oil and cook the ginger, pepper and sprout until a little bit softened. Put the chicken and kale back and add the noodles.
- Tip on the soy, rice wine, lime zest and juice along with enough water to make a sauce that adheres to ingredients, serve straight away.

21. CHICKEN, BROCCOLI AND BEETROOT SALAD WITH AVOCADO PESTO

Prep: 15 Mins, Cook: 15 Mins, Easy Serves: 4

This superfood supper is filled with ingredients to strengthen the body, including red onion, rapeseed oil, nigella seeds, walnuts, and lemon.

Ingredients:

- Thin-strained broccoli, 250gm.
- Rapeseed oil, 2 tsp.
- Three skinless breasts of chicken.
- One red thinly sliced onion.
- Watercress, 100g bag.
- Two raw beetroots (about 175 g), peeled

- Seeds of nigella. 1 tsp.

For pesto avocado.

- Small bag of basil.
- One Avocado.
- Smashed, 1/2 garlic cloves
- Crumbled, 25 g walnut pieces
- Rapeseed oil, 1 tbsp.
- One lemon juice and zest.

Instructions:

- Bring a wide pan of water to a boil, add the broccoli and cook for 2 minutes. Drain, then under cool water to clean. Heat a griddle plate, toss the broccoli for 2-3 mins in 1/2 tsp of the rapeseed oil and griddle, rotating, until a little charred. Put aside to freshen up. Brush the remaining oil and season into the bird. Griddle on either side for 3-4 minutes or until it is cooked clean. Leave to cool, then break into chunky bits or shred them.

- Insert the pesto next. Choose the basil leaves, then set aside a few of them to cover the salad. Place the remainder inside a food processor's little pot. Scoop the avocado flesh and add the garlic, walnuts, sugar, 1 tbsp lemon juice, 2-3 tbsp of cold water and some seasoning to the food processor. Blitz until flat, then move to a small serving platter. Pour the remainder of the lemon juice over the sliced onions, and leave for a few minutes.

- Put the watercress onto a broad bowl. Toss the broccoli and onion, along with the lemon juice in which they were soaked. Top with the beetroot, but don't mix it and the chicken together. Scatter over the reserved basil leaves, the seeds of lemon zest and nigella, then serve with pesto avocado.

22. KALE WITH LEMON TAHINI DRESSING

Prep: 5 Mins, Cook: 5 Mins, Easy   Serves 2

A simple and easy side dish stir-fried on the kale. Drizzle over a glug of the lemon tahini dressing to make your greens flavorful and new

Ingredients:

- One lemon juice (about 3 tbsp)
- Smashed, One garlic clove.
- Tahini, 50 g.
- One cup of olive oil.
- Kale, 200 g.

Instructions:

- In a tiny cup, apply the lemon juice, garlic, tahini and 50ml of cool water. Mix well to form a loose dressing and to taste the seasoning. (Don't panic if it gets divided at first – it should fall back when you mix it).

- Heat the oil in a big pot and stir-fry the kale for 3 minutes. Add half the dressing to the saucepan and cook for 30 secs. Move the remaining dressing to a serving bowl and drizzle over.

23. *THE SIRTFOOD DIET'S CORONATION CHICKEN SALAD*

Easy and safe lunch-spirits

Makes: 1, Prep Time: 0 Hours 5 Mins, COOK TIME: 0 Hours 0 Mins, TOTAL TIME:0 Hours 5 Mins

Ingredients:

- 75 g Yogurt, Regular.
- 1/4 lemon, juiced.
- One tablespoon, chopped, of coriander
- One tablespoon, Turmeric field.
- 1/2 tablespoon of mild curry powder

- 100 g Cooked breast chicken, sliced into bite size

- 6 Half walnut, finely ground.

- 1 Medjool Date, thinly cut.

- 20 g of red onion, Diced.

- 1 bird's eye chili.

- Rocket leaves, 40 grams, for eating

Instructions:

- In a mug, mix the yoghurt, lemon juice, coriander and spices. Attach the remainder of the ingredients and put on a pad of rocket leaves.

24. THE SIRTFOOD DIET'S BUNLESS BEEF BURGERS WITH ALL THE TRIMMINGS

Everybody likes a good burger with sweet fries.

Makes: 1, Prep Time: 0 Hours 15 Mins, Cook Time: 0 Hours 30 Mins, Total Time: 0 Hours 45 Mins

Ingredients:

- 125 g of lean minced beef (5% fat)

- 15 g of red, finely diced onion.

- One tablespoon of Parsley, diced thinly

- 1 tablespoon of Extra virgin Olive oil

- Sweet potatoes, 150 g

- One tablespoon of Olive oil super pure.

- One tablespoon of clean rosemary.

- 1 Clove of garlic, unpeeled.

- 10 gm Cheese cheddar, cut or grated

- 150 g red, ring-sliced onion

- 30 gm Sliced tomato

- Rocket leaves weighing, 10 gm

- One (optional) Gherkin

Instructions:

- Heat the oven up to 220oC / gas 7

- Start by making some fries. Peel and shape the sweet potato into 1 cm thick chips. Attach the olive oil, rosemary and garlic clove to them. Place on a baking sheet and fry for 30 minutes, until smooth and crisp.

- For the steak, combine the ground beef with the onion and the parsley. Unless you have pastry cutters, you may be able to shape your burger with the biggest pastry cutter in the package, otherwise, use your hands to create a decent patty.

- Heat the frying pan over medium heat, add the oil, put the burger patty on one side of the pan and rings the onion on the other side. Cook the patty on each side for 6 minutes, to ensure it is cooked through. When fried to your taste, fry the onion rings.

- Top with the cheese and red onion when the burger patty is cooked and place it in a hot oven for a minute to melt. Top it with the tomato, rocket and gherkin. Serve with some fries.

25. THE SIRTFOOD DIET'S CHICKEN SKEWERS WITH SATAY SAUCE

Dinner with minimal effort, full of taste and spice

Makes: 1, Prep Time: 0 Hours 0 Mins, Cook Time: 0 Hours 0 Mins

Ingredients:

- 150 g of chicken breast, cut into pieces.
- One tablespoon terrestrial turmeric.
- 1/2 tablespoon of Olive oil, particularly virgin.
- Buckwheat: 50 g.
- Kale 30 g, stalks removed and trimmed.
- 30 gm of Sliced celery.
- Four half walnut, sliced, to garnish.
- 20 g of diced red onion
- One Clove of garlic, minced
- One tablespoon of olive oil, particularly virgin
- One tablespoon of curried milk

- One tablespoon of terrestrial turmeric, grated
- Chicken stock: 50 ml
- Coconut milk: 150 ml
- 1 tablespoon butter with walnut or peanut butter
- One tablespoon of chopped Coriander

Instructions:

- Mix the chicken with the turmeric and olive oil and set aside to marinate – 30 minutes to 1 hour would be best, but if you're short on time, just leave it as long as you can.
- Cook the buckwheat according to the package instructions and add the kale and celery for the last 5–7 minutes of the cooking time. Drain.
- Heat the barbecue in a high setting.
- Gently fry the red onion and garlic in the olive oil for 2-3 minutes until soft. Add the spices and cook for another minute. Add the stock and the coconut milk and bring to a boil, then add the walnut butter and stir. Reduce heat and simmer the sauce for 8-10 minutes or until creamy and rich.
- As the sauce simmers, add the chicken to the skewers and place it under the hot grill for 10 minutes, turning it after 5 minutes.
- To serve, stir the coriander in the sauce and pour over the skewers, then spread the chopped walnuts over.

26. THE SIRTFOOD DIET'S SMOKED SALMON OMELETTE

Try this quick and easy Sirtfood dish, packed with taste and goodness.

Makes: 1, Prep Time: 0 Hours 5 Mins, Cook Time: 0 Hours 0 Mins, Total Time: 0 Hours 5 Mins

Ingredients:

- Two eggs small
- 100 g Smoked and cut salmon
- 1/2 dc. Capers
- 10 g of a rocket leaves, cut
- One tablespoon chopped Parsley
- One tablespoon olive oil extra virgin

Instructions:

- Smash the eggs and whisk them into a tub. Stir in the salmon, capers, rockets, and Parsley.
- In a non-stick oven, heat the olive oil till it is dry, but not smoking. Attach the egg blend and push the blend around the pan using a spatula or fish slice until even. Reduce the heat and cook the omelet. Slide around the edges of the spatula and roll the omelet or fold it in half to serve.

27. *THE SIRTFOOD DIET'S SHAKSHUKA*

Enjoy this spicy fried egg and kale recipe.

Makes: 1, Prep Time: 0 Hours 40 Mins, Cook Time: 0 Hours 0 Mins, Total Time: 0 Hours 40 Mins

Ingredients:

- 1 tablespoon of olive Oil, Extra Virgin
- 40 gm of fine cut red onion
- 1 Garlic clove, thinly sliced
- 30 grams of celery, chopped
- 1 bird's eye chili, good cut
- One tablespoon of cumin Ground
- One tablespoon of grated turmeric – Field turmeric.
- One tablespoon of paprika.
- 400 g Chopped tinned tomatoes
- 30 g Kale, trimmed stalks and cut roughly.
- One tablespoon of Parsley.
- Two eggs, small.

Instructions:

- Heat over medium to low heat in a small, deep-seated frying pan. Add the oil and fry onion, garlic, celery, chili, and spices for 1–2 minutes.
- Add the tomatoes, then leave the sauce for 20 minutes to heat slowly, stirring periodically.

28. THE SIRTFOOD DIET'S DATE AND WALNUT PORRIDGE

Get a great start to the day with this Sirtfood breakfast

Makes: 1, Prep Time: 0 Hours 10 Mins, Cook Time: 0 Hours 0 Mins, Total Time: 0 Hours 10 Mins

Ingredients:

- 50 g Strawberries, hulled
- 200 ml Milk or dairy-free alternative
- 35 g Buckwheat flakes
- 1 Medjool date, chopped
- 1 tsp. Walnut butter or four chopped walnut halves

Instructions:

- Put the milk and the date in a saucepan, heat gently, then add the buckwheat flakes and cook until the porridge is the consistency you like.
- Add the walnut butter or walnuts, stir in the strawberries and serve.
- Mix in the kale and roast for another 5 minutes. When you thought the sauce is too thick, just add a bit of water. Stir in the parsley, if your sauce has a good rich flavor.
- Make two small sauce wells and spit each egg into them. Reduce heat to its lowest setting and use a lid or foil to cover the pan. Leave the eggs for 10–12 minutes to cook, where the whites should be firm while the yolks are still runny. Cook for an extra 3–4 minutes, if you like strong yolks. Serve right away-preferably straight from the pan.

29. THE SIRTFOOD DIET'S BRAISED PUY LENTILS

This slow-roasted recipe is full of flavor.

Makes: 1, Prep Time: 0 hours 40 mins, Cook Time: 0 hours 0 mins, Total Time: 0 hours 40 mins

Ingredients:

- 8 Cherry tomatoes, halved
- 40 g Red onion, thinly sliced

- 2 tsp. Extra virgin olive oil

- 40 g Celery, thinly sliced

- 1 Garlic clove, finely chopped

- 1 tsp. Paprika

- 40 g Carrots, peeled and thinly sliced

- 1 tsp. Thyme (dry or fresh)

- 220 ml Vegetable stock

- 75 g Puy lentils

- 20 g Rocket leaves

- 1 tbsp. Parsley, chopped

- 50 g Kale, roughly chopped

Instructions:

- Heat up your oven 120 ° C and gas 1/2 Heat.

- In a small roasting tin, place the tomatoes and roast in the oven for 35-45 minutes.

- Heat the bowl over the medium-low flame. Stir the red Onion, garlic, celery and carrots in 1 teaspoon of olive oil, fry it for 1–2 minutes, until softened. Attach the paprika and thyme and cook for a minute.

- Rinse the lentils and add them to the pot along with the stock in a finely mixed pan. Bring to boil, then raising the heat, cook with a cloth on the saucepan for 20 minutes. Add a little water if the level drops too much and stir every 7 minutes.

- Cook for another 10 minutes, add the kale. Stir in the parsley and roasted tomatoes when the lentils are cooked. Serve the remaining tablespoon with the olive oil with the racket. Serve.

30. THE SIRTFOOD DIET'S PRAWN ARRABBIATA

Ingredients:

- 65 g Buckwheat pasta
- Raw or cooked prawns (Ideally king prawns)
- 1 tbsp. of Extra virgin olive oil
- 1 Garlic clove, finely chopped
- 40 g Red onion, finely chopped
- 1 Bird's eye chili, finely chopped
- 30 g Celery, finely chopped
- 1 tsp. of Dried mixed herbs
- 1 tsp. of Extra virgin olive oil
- 400 g Tinned chopped tomatoes
- 2 tbsp. of White wine (optional)
- 1 tbsp. of Chopped parsley

Instructions:

- Fry the onion, garlic, celery and chili and herbs in oil on half-low heat, for 1-2 minutes. Turn the heat to moderate, add the wine after 1 minute and cook. Attach tomatoes and keep the sauce cooled for 20-30 minutes over medium-low heat until the sauce is nice and creamy. Just add a little water if you feel the sauce is too thick.

- Carry a bowl of water to boil during cooking and cook the pasta as instructed by the packet. Drain and hold in the pan until required.

- Add raw creams to the sauce, cook for 3 to 4 minutes and then add the parsley until they have become rose and opaque, and serve. Bring the sauce to the boil and serve after you have cooked creams with parsley.

- Add cooked pasta to the sauce, carefully yet gently mix and serve.

31. THE SIRTFOOD DIET'S TURMERIC BAKED SALMON

Eastern spices, an easy and healthy dinner.

MAKES: 1, PREP TIME: 0 hours 10 mins, COOK TIME: 0 hours 10 mins, TOTAL TIME: 0 hours 20 mins

Ingredients:

- One tsp. of Ground turmeric
- 2 tsp. Extra virgin olive oil
- 1/4 of a lemon's Juice
- 60 g Tinned green lentils

- 40 g Red onion, finely chopped

- One Bird's eye chili, finely chopped

- One Garlic clove, finely chopped

- One tsp. of Mild curry powder

- 150 gm Celery, cut into 2cm lengths

- 100 ml Chicken or vegetable stock

- 130 gm Tomato, cut into eight wedges

- Skinned Salmon

- One tbsp. Chopped parsley

Instructions:

- Heat the oven to level 6 with gas / 200C.

- Start with the celery and spices. Heat a pot over moderate to low heat, add the onion, garlic, ginger, chili, and celery to 1 tsp of olive oil .. Cook gently until soft and uncolored for about two to three minutes, then add the curry powder and start cooking for another minute.

- Add the tomatoes and the lentils and gently cook for about 10 minutes. You may want to increase or reduce the cooking time according to how crunchy the celery is.

- Mix turmeric, 1 tsp of olive oil and lemon juice in the meantime. Spread mix all over salmon and place on a baking tray. Bake for 8-10 minutes,.

- Finish by mixing the celery with the Parsley and serving with the salmon.

32. EASY PEASY CHICKEN CURRY

Prep Time: 15 minutes, Cook Time: 30 minutes, Total Time: 45 minutes, Servings: 4

Ingredients

- Three garlic cloves, roughly chopped
- One red onion, roughly chopped
- Two teaspoons of garam masala
- 2 cm fresh ginger, peeled and roughly chopped
- Two teaspoons of ground turmeric
- Two teaspoons of ground cumin
- One cinnamon stick, optional
- One tablespoon of olive oil
- Six cardamom pods, optional
- 1 x 400ml tinned coconut milk
- Eight boneless, skinless chicken thighs (or 4 chicken breasts), cut into bitesize chunks
- 200 gm of buckwheat brown rice or basmati rice to serve

- 2 tablespoons of fresh coriander chopped (plus extra for garnish)

Instructions:

- In the food processor, put the onion, garlic and ginger and process until it's a paste. Alternatively, chop these three ingredients thoroughly and continue as below, if you don't have one.

- Stir the garam masala into the paste with cumin and turmeric. Set aside.

- Placed in a big, deep pan (ideally non-stick), 1 tablespoon of olive oil. For a minute, heat up the bowl, then add the chopped chicken thighs. Pour the chicken over a high heat, and add to the curry paste. Turn it down for 2 minutes. Let the chicken cook for 3 minutes in the paste and then add half the milk (200ml) and the cinnamon (if using) as well as the Cardamom. Turn down and cook until the curried sauce is thick and delicious, and then let it simmer for 30 minutes.

- Apply more coconut milk as the curry starts to heat. You may not need anything, but if you want a much more clever curry, add the lot!

- Make your accompaniment (snack / rice) and any side dishes during the cooking process.

- When the curry is finished, add the sliced coriander and serve with sweet or rice and a good glass of white chilled wine or medium water immediately!

33. KING PRAWN STIR FRY WITH BUCKWHEAT NOODLES

Buckwheat Noodles King Prawn Stir Fry

Prep Time: 5 minutes, Cook Time: 15 minutes, Total Time: 20 minutes, Servings: 4

Ingredients:

- 2 tablespoons of extra virgin olive oil
- 300 g buckwheat / soba noodles try to get 100% buckwheat if you can
- 2 sticks of celery, sliced
- 1 red onion, sliced thinly
- 100 g green beans, chopped
- 100 g kale, roughly chopped
- 3 garlic cloves, grated or finely chopped
- 3 cm ginger, grated
- 600 g king prawns
- 1 bird's eye chili seeds/membranes removed and chopped finely (or more to taste)

- 2 tablespoons tamari/soy sauce, plus extra for serving
- 2 tablespoons parsley chopped (or lovage if you can get it!)

Instructions:

- Cook noodles for 3-5 minutes or until you like them. Rinse in cold water, wash. Drizzle over a little olive oil, mix together and set aside.
- Prepare remaining ingredients while the noodles are cooking.
- Fry the red onion and celery in a broad wok or saucepan for 3 minutes in a moderate heat in a mild olive oil and add the kale and green beans and cook for three minutes in medium-high heat.
- Remove heat and add ginger, garlic, chili and butter. Crumble for 2-3 minutes until crevasses are dry.
- Add noodles, tamari / soy sauce, and cook 1 minute longer until the noodles are again dry. Strain and serve with parsley.

34. BAKED POTATOES WITH SPICY CHICKPEA STEW (VEGAN)

Prep Time: 10 minutes, Cook Time: 1 hour, Total Time: 1 hour 10 minutes, Servings: 4 -6

Spicy Chickpea Curry baked potatoes. Mexican mole kind meets North African tagine. It's amazing, makes a perfect top for baked pulp, as well as vegetarian, vegan, gluten free and milk free. And chocolate is there.

Ingredients:

- 2 tablespoons of olive oil
- 4-6 baking potatoes, pricked all over
- 4 cloves garlic, grated or crushed
- 2 red onions, finely chopped
- 2 cm ginger, grated
- 2 tablespoons of cumin seeds
- ½ -2 teaspoons chili flakes, depending on how hot you like things
- A splash of water
- 2 tablespoons of turmeric
- 2 tablespoons unsweetened cocoa powder or cacao
- 2 x 400g tins chickpeas, or kidney beans if you prefer, including the chickpea water. Don't drain!

- 2 yellow peppers or whatever color you prefer!, chopped into bitesize pieces
- 2 x 400g tins chopped tomatoes
- Salt and pepper to taste, optional
- 2 tablespoons of parsley plus extra for garnish
- Side salad optional

Instructions:

- Preheat the oven to 200C, while all the ingredients can be prepared.
- Put potatoes in the oven when the oven is hot enough, and cook for 1 hour or until they're finished as you want them. (If your method is different from mine, feel free to use your usual baked potato method!)
- Put olive oil and chopped red onion in an oven in a big broad casserole in the oven and gradually cook with the lid until the onion is tender, but not brown, for 5 minutes.
- Remove the lid and add the cumin, chili and garlic. Add the curds and a very small splash of water for another minute and cook for a minute, taking care not to let the pan get dry. Cook for a minute.
- Add the tomatoes and cacao powder, chickpeas and yellow pepper, as well as chickpea juice. Bring to a boil, then cook

45 minutes on low heat until the sauce is thick and unctuous (but do not allow it to burn!). The stew will be consumed with the potatoes.

- Serve stewer on the baked potatoes, with a basic side salad, and then add the 2 tablespoons of parsley and salt and pepper if you like.

35. KALE AND RED ONION DHAL WITH BUCKWHEAT (VEGAN)

Kale and Buckwheat Red Onion Dhal. This Kale and Red Onion Dhal is delicious and very nutritious with buckwheat that can be conveniently and quickly processed without gluten, milk, for vegetarians or vegan.

Prep Time: 5 Minutes, Cook Time: 25 Minutes, Total Time: 30 Minutes, Servings4

Ingredients:

- 1 small red onion, sliced
- 1 tablespoon of olive oil
- 2 cm ginger grated
- 3 garlic cloves, grated or crushed
- 2 teaspoons of turmeric

- 1 birds eye chili, deseeded and finely chopped (more if you like things hot!)
- 160 g of red lentils
- 2 teaspoons of garam masala
- 200 ml of water
- 400 ml of coconut milk
- 160 g buckwheat or brown rice
- 100 g kale, or spinach would be a great alternative

Instructions:

• In a deep broad casserole, put the olive oil and add onion, sliced. Cook on low heat, with the lid on so it will be softened for 5 minutes.

• Add garlic, chili ginger and cook for another 1 minute.

• Add the turmeric and a sprinkling of water to the garam masala, and cook for another 1 minute.

• Apply the red lens, chocolate milk and 200 ml of water (just half of the cocoa milk can be filled with water and tipped into the cup).

• Mix everything carefully and cook over low heat with the lid for 20 minutes. Check from time to time, add some more water if the dhal sticks.

• Stir and remove your cap, add a kale after 20 minutes (1-2 minutes if you're using spinach instead!); cook for another 5 minutes.

• Put buckwheat in a medium pot and add plenty of boiling water about 15 minutes before the curry is ready. Return the water to boil again and cook for 10 minutes (or a little longer if it is softer). Drain the buckwheat into a sieve and use the dhal.

36. THE SIRTFOOD DIET GREEN JUICE SALAD

Alternatively to the green sirts, this salad includes two additional Sirt foods, oiled walnuts and olive, with the same ingredients as green juice. Excellent and simple to construct.

Prep Time: 10 Minutes, Total Time: 10 Minutes, Servings1

Ingredients:

- 1 cm ginger, grated
- Juice of ½ a lemon
- 1 tablespoon of olive oil
- Salt and pepper to taste

- 1 handful rocket leaves

- 2 handfuls kale, sliced

- 2 celery sticks, sliced

- 1 tablespoon of parsley

- 6 walnut halves

- ½ green apple, sliced

Instructions:

- In a jam container, add the lemon juice, ginger, salt, pepper and olive oil.

- In a large cup, place the kale and pour over the dressing. Wear the dressing for 1 minute to rub into the kale.

- Add the other ingredients and thoroughly blend together.

37. THE SIRTFOOD DIET GREEN JUICE

The green juice is filled with nutrients-rich Sirt foods, adapted from the recipes in The Sirtfood Diet, which is ideal for anyone who wants a health boost that is important for those following the Sirtfood Diet.

Prep Time: 5 Minutes, Total Time: 5 Minutes, Servings: 1

Ingredients:

- 30 g of rocket leaves
- 75 g of kale
- 5 g of parsley
- ½ a green apple
- 2 celery sticks
- Juice of ½ lemon
- 1 cm of ginger
- ½ teaspoon of matcha green tea

Instructions:

- Juice all the ingredients except the lemon and green tea matcha.
- Set aside the green juice and squeeze the lemon juice.
- Mix in a glass, lemon juice and matcha and add a little green juice. Thoroughly mix and add with the rest of the green juice.
- Save or drink immediately.

38. TURMERIC CHICKEN & KALE SALAD WITH HONEY LIME DRESSING-SIRTFOOD RECIPES

Prep time: 20 mins, Cook time: 10 mins, Total time: 30 mins, Serves: 2

Notes: Dress the salad ten minutes before serving if prepared in advance. Beef small, chopped creeping prawns and fish can replace chicken. Vegetarians may use mushrooms or quinoa cooked.

Ingredients:

For the chicken

- ½ a medium sized brown onion, diced
- 1 teaspoon of ghee or 1 tbsp of coconut oil
- 1 large garlic clove, finely diced
- 250-300 g / 9 oz. chicken mince or diced up chicken thighs
- 1 teaspoon of lime zest
- 1 teaspoon of turmeric powder
- ½ teaspoon of salt + pepper
- juice of ½ lime

For the salad

- 2 tablespoons of pumpkin seeds (pepitas)
- 6 broccolini stalks or 2 cups of broccoli florets
- ½ avocado, sliced
- 3 large kale leaves, stems removed and chopped
- A handful of fresh parsley leaves, chopped
- A handful of fresh coriander leaves, chopped

For the dressing

- 1 small garlic clove, finely diced or grated
- 3 tablespoons of lime juice
- 3 tablespoons of extra-virgin olive oil (I used 1 tablespoons of avocado oil and * 2 tablespoons of EVO)
- 1 teaspoon of raw honey
- 3 tablespoons extra-virgin olive oil (I used 1 tablespoons avocado oil and * 2 tablespoons EVO)
- ½ teaspoon of sea salt and pepper
- ½ teaspoon of wholegrain or Dijon mustard

Instructions:

- In a small frying pan over medium to high flame, heat the ghee or coconut oil. Add onion and sauté 4-5 minutes, until golden, at medium heat. Add the chicken and garlic and turn over medium-high heat for 2-3 minutes and then separate.

- Mix and cook turmeric, lime zest, lime juice, salt and pepper for a further 3-4 minutes . Stir regularly. Put aside the cooked mix.

- Put a small pot of water to boil while the chicken is cooking. Stir and cook the broccolini for 2 minutes. Rinse and cut into 3-4 pieces each under cold water.

- Stirring regularly to avoid burning, add pumpkin seeds into the fry pan from the chicken and toast over medium heat for 2 minutes. Add a little salt seasoning. Season. Set aside. Pure seeds from pumpkin are also appropriate for use.

- In a salad bowl, add the chopped kale and pour over the dressing. Toss the chicken and the dressing with your hands and massage. The humps, like citrus juice to fish or beef carpaccio, are smoothed – they are slightly "cooked."

- Finally add the fried rice, broccolini, new herbs, seeds of pumpkin and avocado.

39. BUCKWHEAT NOODLES WITH CHICKEN KALE & MISO DRESSING-SIRTFOOD RECIPES

Prep time: 15 mins, Cook time: 15 mins, Total time: 30 mins, Serves: 2

Ingredients:

For the noodles

- 2-3 pound of kale leaves (roughly cut from the stem)
- Buckwheat noodles, 150 g/5 oz (100% buckwheat, no wheat)
- 3-4 shiitake champignon, cut..
- 1 tablespoon of ghee or coconut oil.
- 1 brown, fine-diced onion.
- Chicken, sliced or diced, 1 free range breast.
- 1 long, thinly sliced red chili (seeds inside or out, according to how hot you like)
- 2 common, finely diced garlic cloves.
- Tamari sauce with 2-3 teaspoons (gluten-free)

For the miso dressing

- 1 tablespoon of Tamari sauce
- 1½ tablespoon of fresh organic miso
- 1 tablespoon of lemon or lime juice
- 1 tablespoon of extra-virgin olive oil
- 1 teaspoon of sesame oil (optional)

Instructions:

- Put a medium water cup to boil. Add the kale and cook until slightly diluted, for 1 minute. Drain it, and save the water and bring to boil again. Fill with the soba noodles and cook (usually approximately 5 minutes) according to package directions. Rinse and set aside under cold water.

- Meanwhile, fry the shiitake champignon for 2-3 minutes with a little ghee or coconut oil (around a teaspoon), until nicely browned on either side. Sprinkle in salt and set aside..

- Heat coconut oil or ghee over medium-high heat in the same frying saucepan. Pour in onion and chili and add chicken parts for 2-3 minutes. Cook over medium heat five minutes, stirring a few times, then add a small amount of garlic, tamari sauce, and tea. Cook for another 2-3 minutes, mix frequently until chicken is done.

- Add the chicken noodle and soba, and mix in the food on heat.

- Just before taking it off the heat, blend the miso dressing and twinkling over the noodles to keep all of these beneficial probiotics alive.

40. CHOC CHIP GRANOLA-SIRTFOOD RECIPES

244 calories, 1/2 of your SIRT 5 a day, Serves 8, Ready in 30 minutes

Breakfast cake! Make sure to serve yourself plenty of SIRTs with a cup of green tea. If you want, you can substitute the rice malt syrup with maple syrup.

Ingredients:

- 50g pecans, roughly chopped
- 200g jumbo oats
- 20g butter
- 3 tbsp of light olive oil
- 2 tbsp of rice malt syrup
- 1 tbsp of dark brown sugar
- 60g good-quality (70%) dark chocolate chips

Instructions

- Preheat oven to 140 ° C (gas 3). • Preheat oven to 160 ° C. Line a major bakery with a sheet of silicone or pastry.

- In a large pan, mix oats and pecans. Heat olive oil, butter, brown sugar and rice malt syrup gently in a small, non-stick pot separately until butter melts and the sugar and syrup are dissolved. Don't heat with oat mix. Pour the syrup over the oats and mix until the oats fully covered.

- Spread the granola in a baking pan and spread into the corners. Having mixture clumps with distance instead of spreading. Leave for twenty minutes in the oven until the edges are light brown. Take out of the oven and allow the tray to completely refresh.

- Separate with your fingertips and then blend with the chocolate chips with any large clumps in a tray when it's cold. Grab or pour the granola into a bowl or container airtight. The granola will stay for at least 2 weeks.

41. BAKED SALMON SALAD WITH CREAMY MINT DRESSING-SIRTFOOD RECIPES

340 Calories, 3 Of Your SIRT 5 A Day, Serves 1, Ready In 20 Minutes

It's quick to roast the salmon in the oven.

Ingredients:

- 40g of mixed salad leaves
- 1 salmon fillet (130g)
- 2 radishes, trimmed and thinly sliced
- 40g of young spinach leaves
- 2 spring onions, trimmed and sliced
- 5cm piece (50g) of cucumber, cut into chunks
- 1 small handful (10g) of parsley, roughly chopped

For the dressing:

- 1 tbsp of natural yogurt
- 1 tsp of low-fat mayonnaise
- 2 leaves mint, finely chopped
- 1 tbsp of rice vinegar
- Salt and freshly ground black pepper

Instructions:

- Preheat the oven to 200C (fan / gas 6 at a temperature of 180C).
- Put the salmon fillet on a baking pan and bake until cooked, for 16-18 minutes. Remove and set aside from the oven. The salmon in the salad will be just as nice warm or cold. If your salmon has a lot of meat, just cook with the skin downwards

and separate it from the skin with a fish slice. When cooked, it will slide off quickly.

- Mix the mayonnaise, yoghurt and rice vinegar together in a small bowl and add the mint leaves, salt and pepper to the mixture to allow the aromas to develop for at least 5 minutes.
- Set the mixed salad leaves and spinach with radishes, cucumber, spring onions and parsley on the serving plate and top. Place the cooked salmon on the salad and dressing on top.

42. FRAGRANT ASIAN HOTPOT-SIRTFOOD RECIPES

185 Calories, 1 1/2 Of You SIRT 5 A Day, Serves 2, Ready In 15 Minutes

Ingredients:

- 1 star anise, crushed (or 1/4 tsp ground anise)
- 1 tsp of tomato purée
- Small handful (1Og) of coriander, stalks finely chopped
- Small handful (10g) of parsley, stalks finely chopped
- 1/2 a carrot, peeled and cut into matchsticks
- 50g beansprouts
- 50g broccoli, cut into small florets
- 100g firm tofu, chopped

- 100g raw tiger prawns

- 50g rice noodles, cooked according to packet

- 20g sushi ginger, chopped

- 50g cooked water chestnuts, drained

- 1 tbsp good-quality miso paste

Instructions:

- Put in broad pan and simmer for 10 minutes, the stir in the tomato, star anise, petty stalks, coriander stalks and lime juice.

- Add carrot, broccoli, creeping pies, tofu, chestnuts and rice noodles and gently cook, until creeping is finished. Stir in the sushi ginger and miso paste once removed from the heat .

- Serve with parsley and coriander leaves. Sprinkle serving.

43. LAMB,BUTTERNUT SQUASH AND DATE TAGINE-SIRTFOOD RECIPES

Prep Time: 15 Mins, Cook Time: 1 Hour 15 Mins, Total Time: 1 Hour 30 Mins, Serves: 4

Unbelievable dry Moroccan spices make this balanced day ideal for icy fall and winter days. For an extra health kick, serve with buckwheat!

Ingredients:

- 1 red onion, sliced
- 2 tablespoons of olive oil
- 3 garlic cloves, grated or crushed
- 2cm ginger, grated
- 2 teaspoons of cumin seeds
- 1 teaspoon of chili flakes (or to taste)
- 2 teaspoons of ground turmeric
- 1 cinnamon stick
- ½ teaspoon of salt
- 800g lamb neck fillet, cut into 2cm chunks
- 500g butternut squash, chopped into 1cm cubes
- 400g tin chopped tomatoes, plus half a can of water
- 2 tablespoons fresh coriander (plus extra for garnish)
- 400g tin chickpeas, drained
- Buckwheat, couscous, flatbreads or rice to serve

Instructions:

- Preheat to 140C for your oven.
- Drizzle two tablespoons of olive oil in a large ovenproof casserole dish. Slice onion and heat until the onions are smooth but not browned, with a cover on for about 5 minutes.

- Ginger, garlic chili, cumin, cinnamon, and turmeric should be added in . Cover well and cook with the lid for another 1 minute. If it gets too dry, add a sprinkle of water.

- Add next, chunks of lamb. Add the butter, minced dates and tomato and a further half a can of water (100-200mL) to cover the meat in the onions and Spices. Mix well.

- Bring the tagine to a simmer, then place on the cover and place 1 hour and 15 minutes in your pre-heated oven.

- Add chopped butternut squash and drained chickpeas thirty minutes prior to the end of the cooking period. Put the cover on and back in the oven for the remaining 30 minutes of the preparation, bringing it together.

- Turn off the oven and mix with chopped coriander when tagine is finished. Serve with couscous, basmati or buckwheat.

Notes

If you don't own an ovenproof casserole or iron cast casserole dish, just bake the tagine in an ordinary bowl until it's in the oven and transfer it to an ordinary saucer before putting the tagine in the oven. Add an additional five minutes to cook to give more room to heat in the saucepan.

44. PRAWN ARRABBIATA-SIRTFOOD RECIPES

Serves 1, Preparation Time: 35 – 40 Minutes, Cooking Time: 20 – 30 Minutes

Ingredients:

- 65 g of Buckwheat pasta
- 125-150 g of Raw or cooked prawns (Ideally king prawns)
- For arrabbiata sauce
- 1 tbsp of Extra virgin olive oil
- 1 Garlic clove, finely chopped
- 40 g Red onion, finely chopped
- 1 Bird's eye chili, finely chopped
- 30 g of Celery, finely chopped
- 1 tsp of Extra virgin olive oil
- 1 tsp of Dried mixed herbs
- 400 g of Tinned chopped tomatoes
- 2 tbsp of White wine (optional)
- 1 tbsp of Chopped parsley

Instructions:

- Fry in oil on a half-low heat, for 1-2 minutes the onion, garlic, celery and chili and herbs. Switch the heat to mild, add the wine for 1 minute and cook. Add tomatoes and keep the sauce cooled for 20-30 minutes over medium-low heat until the sauce is good and thick. Just add a little water if you feel the sauce is too thick.

- Bring a bowl of water to boil during cooking and cook the pasta as directed by the packet. Drain the olive oil and keep in the pan until necessary.

- Add raw creams to the sauce, cook for 3 to 4 minutes and then add the parsley until they have become rose and opaque, and serve. Allow the sauce to the boil.

- Add to the sauce cooked pasta, carefully but gently mix and serve.

45. TURMERIC BAKED SALMON SIRTFOOD RECIPES

Serves: 1, Preparation Time: 10 – 15 Minutes, Cooking Time: 10 Minutes

Ingredients:

- 1 tsp of Extra virgin olive oil
- 125-150 g of Skinned Salmon
- 1/4 Juice of a lemon
- 1 tsp of Ground turmeric

- 1 tsp of Extra virgin olive oil

For the spicy celery

- 60 g of Tinned green lentils
- 40 g Red onion, finely chopped
- 1 cm of Fresh ginger, finely chopped
- 1 Garlic clove, finely chopped
- 150 g of Celery, cut into 2cm lengths
- 1 Bird's eye chili, finely chopped
- 130 g of Tomato, cut into 8 wedges
- 1 tsp of Mild curry powder
- 1 tbsp of Chopped parsley
- 100 ml of Chicken or vegetable stock

Instructions:

- Heat the furnace to 200C / gas 6.
- Coat the pot with olive oil, then add onion, garlic, ginger, chili and celery over low-medium flame. Fritter gently for 2 to 3 minutes and then apply the curry powder and cook for another minute, until softer but not marked.
- Then add the tomatoes and the lentils and gently cook for 10 minutes. You might want to increase or reduce the cooking time according to how crunchy the celery is.

- Mix the turmeric, butter and lemon juice in the meantime, then roll the salmon over it. Place on the baking tray, bake for 8-10 minutes,.
- Stir in celery and serve with the salmon to finish.

46. CORONATION CHICKEN SALAD

Serves 1, Preparation Time: 5 Minutes

Ingredients:

- Juice of 1/4 of a lemon
- 75 g of Natural yoghurt
- 1 tsp of Ground turmeric
- 1 tsp of Coriander, chopped
- 100 g of Cooked chicken breast, cut into bite-sized pieces
- 1/2 tsp of Mild curry powder
- 1 Medjool date, finely chopped
- 6 Walnut halves, finely chopped
- 1 Bird's eye chili
- 20 g of Red onion, diced
- 40 g of Rocket leaves, to serve

Instruction:

- In a cup, mix the milk, the lemon juice, coriander and the spices. Serve on a rocket leaves bed, adding all remaining ingredients.

47. BAKED POTATOES WITH SPICY CHICKPEA STEW-SIRTFOOD RECIPES

Prep Time: 10 Mins, Cook Time: 1 Hour, Serves 4-6

A sort of Mexican Mole, this Hot STEW TREE is amazingly wonderful and offers an outstanding topping with baked potatoes plus its vegetarian, organic, gluten-free and milk-free. And chocolate is in it.

Ingredients:

- 2 tablespoons of olive oil
- 4-6 baking potatoes, pricked all over
- 4 cloves of garlic, grated or crushed
- 2 red onions, finely chopped
- ½ -2 teaspoons of chili flakes (depending on how hot you like things)
- 2cm of ginger, grated
- 2 tablespoons of turmeric
- 2 tablespoons of cumin seeds

- 2 x 400g tins of chopped tomatoes

- Splash of water

- 2 x 400g tins of chickpeas (or kidney beans if you prefer) including the chickpea water DON'T DRAIN!!

- 2 tablespoons of unsweetened cocoa powder (or cacao)

- 2 tablespoons of parsley plus extra for garnish

- Salt and pepper to taste (optional)

- 2 yellow peppers (or whatever color you prefer!), chopped into bitesize pieces

- Side salad (optional)

Instructions:

- Preheat the oven to 200C.

- Place the baking potatoes in the oven when the oven is high enough, and cook for 1 hour or until they're cooked as you want them.

- Put olive oil and sliced red onion in an oven in a big broad casserole once in the oven and gradually cook with the cover until the onion is tender, but not brown for 5 minutes.

- Remove the cover and apply the cumin, chili and garlic. Add the curds and a very tiny splash of water and cook for another minute, take care not to make the pan hot unnecessarily. Cook for a minute.

- Introduce the tomatoes and cacao powder, chickpeas and yellow pepper, as well as chickpea juice. Bring to a boil, then cook for 45 minutes on low heat until the sauce is thick and unctuous (but do not let it burn!). The stew will eaten with the potatoes.

- Put a stewer on the baked potatoes, with a basic side salad, and then apply the 2 teaspoons of parsley and salt and pepper if you want.

48. GRAPE AND MELON JUICE-SIRTFOOD RECIPES

125 Calories, 2 Of Your Sirt 5 A Day, Serves: 1, Ready In 2 Minutes

Ingredients:

- 1/2 cucumber, peel if necessary, halving, scraping seeds and roughing.
- 30 g youthful spinach leaves, removed stalks.
- 100 g red grapes without seeds.
- 100 g of melon, washed, wished and cut cantaloupe.

Instruction:

- In a juicer or blender, mix everything together until smooth.

49. KALE AND RED ONION DHAL WITH BUCKWHEAT

Prep Time: 5 Mins, Cook Time: 25 Mins, Total Time: 30 Mins, Serves:4

This Kale and Red Onion Dhal is tasty and very healthy with a buckwheat that can be conveniently and rapidly processed without gluten or oil, for vegetarians or vegan.

Ingredients:

- 1 small red onion, sliced
- 1 tablespoon of olive oil
- 2 cm of ginger, grated
- 3 garlic cloves, grated or crushed
- 2 teaspoons of turmeric
- 1 birds eye chili, deseeded and finely chopped (more if you like things hot!)
- 160g of red lentils
- 2 teaspoons of garam masala
- 200ml of water
- 400ml of coconut milk
- 160g of buckwheat (or brown rice)
- 100g of kale (or spinach would be a great alternative)

Instructions:

- In a broad deep casserole, apply the olive oil and dice the onion into it. Cook in low temperatures with the lid until softened, for 5 minutes.
- Add garlic, ginger and chili, and fry.
- Apply turmeric, garam masala and splash water and cook 1 minute more.
- Fill in red lentils, coconut milk and 200ml of water, the coconut milk may be loaded with water and tipped into the bowl.
- Thoroughly mix and cook over medium heat with the lid on for 20 minutes. Remove from time to time, add a little more water when the dhal stays.
- Add the kale and mix carefully.
- Cook for another 5 minutes (1-2 minutes if using spinach instead)
- Put buckwheat in a medium pot and add plenty of boiling water about 15 minutes before the curry is finished.
- Take your buckwheat back on heat to boil and cook it for 10 minutes, or for a little bit longer if you like your softer buckwheat.

50. CHARGRILLED BEEF WITH A RED WINE JUS, ONION RINGS, GARLIC KALE AND HERB ROASTED POTATOES-SIRTFOOD RECIPES

Ingredients:

- 1 tbsp of extra virgin olive oil
- 100g potatoes, peeled and cut into 2cm dice
- 50g red onion, sliced into rings
- 5g parsley, finely chopped
- 1 garlic clove, finely chopped
- 50g kale, sliced
- 40ml of red wine
- 120–150g x 3.5cm-thick beef fillet steak or 2cm-thick sirloin steak
- 1 tsp of tomato purée
- 150ml of beef stock
- 1 tsp of corn flour, dissolved in 1 tbsp water

Instructions:

- Oven power to 220 ° C / gas 7.
- Place the potatoes in a boiling pot and then drain for 4–5 minutes and put back to boil. In a roasting pan, apply 1 tablespoon of olive oil and roast for 35-45 minutes in the hot oven. Place the potatoes in order to ensure an even cooking

for 10 minutes. Sprinkle the chopped parsley and mix well when cooked from the oven.

- Fry onion for 5 to 7 minutes in one teaspoon of oil until soft and beautifully caramelized over medium heat. Keep dry. Keep it warm. Steam the kale and drain for about 2-3 minutes. Cook the goat softly, but not colored, in 1/2 teaspoon of oil for 1 minute. Add the kale and onion for another 1–2 minutes.

- Leave a high-heat oven-proof frying pan to smoke. Cook the meat in 1/2 teaspoon of oil and mix in the heated bowl over medium-high flame, if you prefer your beef very tender. If you want to use the beef mild, stitch the meat and move the bowl to a 220oC / gas 7 furnace, such that the cooking may be done for the specified periods.

- Take the meat out of the pot and put it aside. To collect any residue of meat, add wine to the hot pot. Let bubble for a balanced taste.

- Add the pan to the steaked bowl, the tomato puree and the corn flour paste and thicken the sauce until you are sure of the perfect consistency. Add the carrots, onions, onion rings and red sauce in the relaxed steak juice and eat.

51. KALE AND BLACKCURRANT SMOOTHIE-SIRTFOOD RECIPES

86 calories, 1 – 1/2 of your SIRT 5 a day, Serves: 2, Ready in 3 minutes

Ingredients:

- 1 cup freshly made green tea
- 2 tsp of honey
- 1 ripe banana
- 10 baby kale leaves, stalks removed
- 6 ice cubes
- 40 g of blackcurrants, washed and stalks removed

Instructions:

- Extract the honey until it is absorbed in the dry, green tea. Mix all ingredients into a fast food processor or blender. Serve immediately.

52. BUCKWHEAT PASTA SALAD-SIRTFOOD RECIPES

Serves 1

Instructions:

- large handful of rocket leaves
- 50g buckwheat pasta (cooked according to the packet instructions)Sirtfood recipes
- 8 cherry tomatoes, halved
- small handful of basil leaves
- 10 olives
- 1/2 avocado, diced
- 20g of pine nuts
- 1 tbsp of extra virgin olive oil

Instructions:

- Mix all ingredients gently with the exception of the pine nut, and then arrange them on a plate or in a bowl. And add pine nuts.

53. GREEK SALAD SKEWERS

306 calories, 3.5 of your SIRT 5 a day, Serves: 2, Ready in 10 minutes

Ingredients:

- 8 large black olives
- 2 wooden skewers, soaked in water for 30 minutes before use
- 1 yellow pepper, cut into 8 squares
- 8 cherry tomatoes
- 100g (about 10cm) of cucumber, cut into 4 slices and halved
- ½ red onion, cut in half and separated into 8 pieces
- 100g feta, cut into 8 cubes

For the dressing:

- Juice of ½ a lemon
- 1 tbsp of extra virgin olive oil
- ½ clove of garlic, peeled and crushed
- 1 tsp of balsamic vinegar
- Few oregano leaves, finely chopped
- Few basil leaves, finely chopped (or ½ tsp dried mixed herbs to replace basil and oregano)
- Generous seasoning of salt and freshly ground black pepper

Instructions:

- Thread ingredients per skewer in this order for the salad: olive, tomato, red onion, cucumber, cucumber, basil, garlic, red onion, pepper, feta.
- In a small pot, put all the dressing components and combine thoroughly together. Verse the skewers around.
- Serve salad skewers with dressing

54. KALE, EDAMAME AND TOFU CURRY-SIRTFOOD RECIPES

342 calories, 2 1/2 of your SIRT 5 a day

Warm curry and winter curry. Simple to hold cooled or frozen for another day.

Serves: 4, Ready in 45 minutes

Ingredients:

- 1 large onion, chopped
- 1 tbsp of rapeseed oil
- 1 large thumb (7cm) of fresh ginger, peeled and grated
- 4 cloves of garlic, peeled and grated

- 1/2 tsp of ground turmeric
- 1 red chili, deseeded and thinly sliced
- 1 tsp of paprika
- 1/4 tsp of cayenne pepper
- 1 tsp of salt
- 1/2 tsp of ground cumin
- 1 liter boiling water
- 250g of dried red lentils
- 200g of firm tofu, chopped into cubes
- 50g frozen soya edamame beans
- Juice of 1 lime
- 2 tomatoes, roughly chopped
- 200g of kale leaves, stalks removed and torn

Instructions

- Place the oil in a heavy-bottom pan over low-medium sun. Add the onion and cook for 5 minutes before inserting the garlic, ginger and chili, and cook for another 2 minutes. Remove the chili, cayenne, paprika, cumin and oil. Swirl once before inserting the red lentils and swirl again.
- Pour in boiling water and simmer for 10 minutes, then raise the heat and cook for another 20-30 minutes so the curry has a deep '•porridge' consistency.

- Add the rice, tofu and tomatoes and simmer for another 5 minutes. Add the lime juice and the kale leaves, then cook until the kale is soft.

55. CHOCOLATE CUPCAKES WITH MATCHA ICING-SIRTFOOD RECIPES

234 calories, 1 of your SIRT 5 a day, MAKES 12, READY IN 35 MINUTES

Ingredients:

- 200g of caster sugar
- 150g of self-raising flour
- ½ tsp of salt
- 60g of cocoa
- 120 ml of milk
- ½ tsp of fine espresso coffee, decaf if preferred
- 50ml of vegetable oil
- ½ tsp of vanilla extract
- 120ml of boiling water
- 1 egg

For the icing:

- 50g of icing sugar
- 50g of butter, at room temperature
- ½ tsp of vanilla bean paste
- 1 tbsp of matcha green tea powder
- 50g of soft cream cheese

Instructions:

- Preheat the oven to a fan of 180C/160C. Cover a cupcake tray with a paper or silicone cake shell.

- Place the rice, sugar, chocolate, salt and espresso powder in a large bowl and blend thoroughly.

- Apply the cream, vanilla extract, vegetable oil and egg with the dry ingredients and use an electric mixer until well mixed. Carefully dump in the boiling water gradually and mix at low speed before fully mixed. Using high speed to beat for another minute and add speed to the pump. The batter will be even more oily than the normal cake blend. Have faith, it's going to taste amazing!

- Pour the batter equally between the cake cases. Each case of a cake will not be more than 3/4 full. Bake in the oven for 15-18 minutes, before the mixture has been tapped out. Remove from the oven and allow it to cool completely before icing.

- Mix the butter and icing sugar together until it is light and creamy. Add the matcha powder and vanilla, stir again. Attach the cream cheese and beat until smooth. Pipe or spray it over the cakes.

56. SESAME CHICKEN SALAD

Serve 2, ready in 12 minute 304 cals, 3.5 your SIRT 5 a day

A delicious and unusual salad.

Ingredients:

- 1 cucumber, peeled, halved lengthways, deseeded with a teaspoon and sliced
- 1 tbsp of sesame seeds
- 60g pak choi, very finely shredded
- 100g of baby kale, roughly chopped
- Large handful (20g) parsley, chopped
- ½ red onion, very finely sliced
- 150g of cooked chicken, shredded

For the dressing:

- 1 tsp of sesame oil
- 1 tbsp of extra virgin olive oil
- 1 tsp of clear honey
- Juice of 1 lime
- 2 tsp of soy sauce

Instructions:

- Toast seeds of sesame in a gently browned and fragrant saucepan for 2 minutes. Move to a cooling pad.

- Mix olive oil, sesame oil, lime juice, sweet honey, and soy sauce together in a small bowl for the dressing.

- In a big pot, heat the cucumber, the kale, the choi box, the red onion, and the peanut. Place the dressing on and mix again.

- Distribute the salad to the top of the chicken and between two plates. Just before eating, scatter the sesame seeds over.

57. MUSHROOM SCRAMBLE EGGS

Ingredients:

- 1 tsp over ground turmeric
- 2 eggs
- 20g over kale, roughly chopped
- 1 tsp over mild curry powder
- ½ bird's eye chili, thinly sliced
- 1 tsp over extra virgin olive oil
- 5g over parsley, finely chopped
- A handful of button mushrooms (Champignons), thinly sliced
- Add a seed mixture as a topper and some Rooster Sauce for flavor (Optional)

Instructions:

- Mix curry powder and turmeric and apply a little water until a soft paste is achieved.
- Add eggs and parsley to curry mix and beat together.
- Steam the kale for two to three minutes.
- In a frying pan, heat oil over medium heat and fry the chilies and champignons for 2-3 minutes until browned and sweetened.

- Add egg mixture to champignon and gently stir mixture until eggs are thickened and no liquid egg remains, for a couple of minutes.

- Add Kale, allow to cook for 1 minute. Top with seed mixture and serve.

58. AROMATIC CHICKEN BREAST WITH KALE, RED ONION, AND SALSA

Ingredients:

- 2 tsp of ground turmeric
- 120g of skinless, boneless chicken breast
- 1 tbsp of extra virgin olive oil
- juice of ¼ lemon
- 20g of red onion, sliced
- 50g of kale, chopped
- 50g of buckwheat
- 1 tsp chopped fresh ginger

Instructions:

- To produce the salsa, cut the eye from the tomato and finely slice to take sure that the liquid is retained as much as possible. Mix chili, capers, lemon juice and parsley together.

You should place it all in a blender, but the effects are somewhat different.

- Oven power to 220 ° C / gas 7. Mix 1 tablespoon of the turmeric, the lemon juice and a little oil to marinate the chicken breast. For 5–10 minutes.

- Heat an oven resistant pot till it's hot, then add the marinated chicken and cook on all sides for a minute or more, until pale golden, then move to the oven for 8–10 minutes (place on the baking tray if your pot is not stove resistant). Take from the oven, cover with foil and give 5 minutes to rest before serving.

- Cook the kale for 5 minutes in a steamer. With a little olive oil, fry the red onions and the ginger until they are tender, though not cooked.

- Cook the buckwheat with the remaining tablespoon of turmeric in compliance with the package directions. Serve with chicken, greens and salsa.

59. SMOKED SALMON OMELETTE

Try this quick and easy Sirtfood platter full of goodness and flavor.

Serves: 1, Preparation time: 5 – 10 minutes

Ingredients:

- 100 g of Smoked salmon, sliced
- 2 Medium eggs
- 10 g of Rocket leaves, chopped
- 1/2 tsp of Capers
- 1 tsp of Extra virgin olive oil
- 1 tsp of Parsley, chopped

Instructions:

- Rub the eggs and whisk them in a bowl. Stir in tuna, shells, rocket leaves and peanuts.
- In a non-stick frying pan, heat the olive oil to steam but not to burn. Add the mixture and move the mixture around the pan until it is even with a spatula or fish slice. Reduce the fire and prepare the omelet. Run along the sides of the spatula and roll up or fold the omelet to slice in half.

60. GREEN TEA SMOOTHIE

183 calories, 1 of your SIRT 5 a day, Serves: 2, Ready in 3 minutes

This super healthy smoothie uses an extremely enriched Japanese green tea blended with matcha powder. It is accessible in Asian specialists or in tea shops.

Ingredients:

- 250 of ml milk
- 2 ripe bananas
- 1/2 tsp of vanilla bean paste (not extract) or a small scrape of the seeds from a vanilla pod
- 2 tsp of matcha green tea powder
- 2 tsp of honey
- 6 ice cubes

Instructions:

- Simply mix every ingredient together in a mixer, processor or blender and serve in two cups.

61. SIRT FOOD MISO MARINATED COD WITH STIR FRIED GREENS & SESAME SIRT-FOOD RECIPES

Serves 1

Ingredients:

- 1 tbsp of mirin
- 20g miso
- 200g of skinless cod fillet
- 1 tbsp of extra virgin olive oil
- 40g of celery, sliced
- 20g red onion, sliced
- 1 bird's eye chili, finely chopped
- 1 garlic clove, finely chopped
- 60g green beans
- 1 tsp of finely chopped fresh ginger
- 1 tsp of sesame seeds
- 50g kale, roughly chopped
- 1 tbsp of tamari
- 5g parsley, roughly chopped
- 1 tsp of ground turmeric
- 30g buckwheat

Instructions:

- Mix the miso, mirin and 1 teaspoon of olive oil. Clean the entire cod, apply mix and set for 30 minutes to marinate. To 220oC / gas fire the oven to 7.

- 10 minutes to bake cod.

- Heat a wide frying bowl in the meantime or wok with the rest of the oil. Add the celery, garlic, curry, ginger, green beans, and kale, then leave it for a few minutes. Tender fry until it is cooked. To help the cooking phase you can have to apply a little water to the oven.

- Cook the buckwheat with the turmeric for 3 minutes according to the package directions.

- Serve in a stir fry with greens and shrimp, incorporate sesame seeds, parsley, tamari.

62. RASPBERRY AND BLACKCURRANT JELLY-SIRTFOOD RECIPES

76 calories, 2 SIRT 5 per day, Serves: 2, ready 15 minutes + time set

Jelly-making is an ideal way to prepare the fruit such that it's able to consume in the morning for the first time.

Instructions:

- Two leaves of gelatin, Sirtfood recipes
- 100g raspberries, washed

- Two tbsp of granulated sugar

- 100gm blackcurrants, washed and stalks removed

- 300ml of water

Instructions:

- Arrange in two dishes / glasses / mold the raspberries. In a bowl of cold water, soften the gelatin leaves.

- Put in sugar and 100ml of water and use to boil the blackcurrants in a small pot. Drop into the fire and whisk vigorously for five minutes. Wait for two minutes.

- Spray the gelatin leaves with extra water and add it to the pot. Add the remaining water until it is dissolved. Put the fluid in the cooked plates and cool to set. In 3-4 hours or overnight, the jellies should be set.

63. APPLE PANCAKES WITH BLACKCURRANT COMPOTE-SIRTFOOD RECIPES

337 calories, 1 1/2 of you SIRT 5 a day, Serves 4 • Ready in 20 minutes

These pancakes are healthy and decadent. A lovely morning dish.

Instructions:

- 75g of porridge oats
- 2 tbsp of caster sugar
- 1 tsp of baking powder
- 125g plain flour
- 2 apples, peeled, cored and cut into small pieces
- Pinch of salt
- 2 egg whites
- 300ml of semi-skimmed milk
- 2 tsp of light olive oil

For the compote:

- 2 tbsp of caster sugar
- 120g of blackcurrants, washed and stalks removed
- 3 tbsp of water

Instructions:

- Make the compote first. Put the blackcurrants, sugar and water in a small saucepan. Bring to a burner and boil for 10-15 minutes.

- In a wide pot, put the oats, flour, baking powder, caster sugar and salt and mix well. Stir in the apple and whisk in the milk a little at a time until you have a smooth blend. Whisk the egg whites to firm peaks, then insert into the batter for the pancake. Put the batter over to a jug.

- Heat 1/2 tsp of oil over medium-high heat in a non-stick frying pan and dump around one fourth of the batter into it. Cook until light brown, on all sides. Do same for the four pancakes and repeat to make.

- Eat the pancakes drizzled over with blackcurrant compote.

64. FRUIT SALAD

172 cal, 3 of your SIRT 5 a day, Serves: 1, Ready in 10 minutes

This fruit salad is filled with the finest SIRT fruits.

Ingredients:

- 1 tsp of honey
- ½ cup of freshly made green tea
- 1 apple, cored and roughly chopped
- 1 orange, halved

- 10 blueberries

- 10 red seedless grapes

Instructions:

- Stir in half a cup of green tea with the sugar. When diluted, add the half orange juice. Leave on to cool down.

- Cut the other half of the orange and put the sliced fruit, grapes and blueberries together in a dish. Pour over the cooled tea, and leave to steep before serving for a few minutes.

65. BITES-SIRTFOOD RECIPES

Ingredients

- 30g of dark chocolate (85 per cent cocoa solids), broken into pieces; or cocoa nibs

- 120g of walnuts

- 1 tbsp of cocoa powder

- 250g Medjool dates, pitted

- 1 tbsp of extra virgin olive oil

- 1 tbsp of ground turmeric

- 1–2 tbsp of water

- the scraped seeds of one vanilla pod or 1 tsp of vanilla extract

Instructions:

- In a food processor, place the walnuts and chocolate and process them until they make a fine powder.

- Add all the remaining ingredients except water and combine until the mixture forms a disk. Depending on the strength of the paste, you may or do not have to apply the water-you don't want it to be so wet.

- Shape the mixture into bite-sized balls with your hands and refrigerate in an airtight jar for at least one hour prior to feeding.

- Add in some more chocolate or desiccated cocoa, you could roll any of the balls to obtain a different finish if you want.

- They'll stay in your fridge for up to one week.

66. SIRT MUESLI-SIRTFOOD RECIPES

Ingredients:

- 10g of buckwheat puffs
- 20g of buckwheat flakes Sirtfood recipes
- 40g of Medjool dates, pitted and chopped
- 15g of coconut flakes or desiccated coconut
- 10g of cocoa nibs
- 15g of walnuts, chopped
- 100g of plain Greek yoghurt (or vegan alternative, such as soya or coconut yoghurt)

- 100g of strawberries, hulled and chopped

Instructions:

- Mix all of the above ingredients together and incorporate yogurt and strawberries only when you mixed them in bulk, before serving.

67. CHINESE-STYLE PORK WITH PAK CHOI-SIRTFOOD RECIPES

377 CALORIES AND 2 OF YOUR SIRT 5 A DAY, Serves: 4

Ingredients:

- 1 tbsp of corn flour Sirtfood recipes
- 400g of firm tofu, cut into large cubes
- 125ml of chicken stock
- 1 tbsp of water
- 1 tbsp of tomato purée
- 1 tbsp of rice wine
- 1 tbsp of soy sauce
- 1 tsp of brown sugar
- 1 thumb (5cm) of fresh ginger, peeled and grated 1 tbsp rapeseed oil
- 1 clove garlic, peeled and crushed

- 1 shallot, peeled and sliced

- 100g of shiitake mushrooms, sliced

- 100g of beansprouts

- 200g of pak choi or choi sum, cut into thin slices 400g pork mince (10% fat)

- Large handful (20g) of parsley, chopped

Instructions:

- Lay tofu on paper in the kitchen, cover with more paper for the kitchen and set aside.

- Combine the corn flour with water and scrape all the lumps together in a shallow tub. Stir in the onions, rice vinegar, puree onion, brown sugar and soy sauce. Stir together the moved garlic and ginger.

- Heat oil to high temperature in a wok or wide frying pan. Add the shiitake mushrooms and fry until shiny and brightened for 2–3 minutes. Take out the mushrooms and set back. Add tofu to the saucepan and turn until golden everywhere. Enter and put aside by using a slotted spoon.

- Stir-fry in the wok for two minutes and then substitute the thin choi. Cook until the thin choi has been fried, then add the sauce, reduce the heat for one minute or two and allow the sauce to bubble around the beef. Throw the breadcrumbs, shiitake champignon and tofu into the pan and add a bit of water. Remove it from the flame, detach it and instantly drink.

68. TUSCAN BEAN STEW-SIRTFOOD RECIPES

Ingredients:

- 50g of red onion, finely chopped
- 1 tbsp of extra virgin olive oil
- 30g of celery, trimmed and finely chopped
- 30g of carrot, peeled and finely chopped
- ½ bird's eye chili, finely chopped (optional)
- 1 garlic clove, finely chopped
- 200ml of vegetable stock
- 1 tsp of herbes de Provence
- 1 tsp of tomato purée
- 1 x 400g of tin chopped Italian tomatoes
- 50g of kale, roughly chopped
- 200g of tinned mixed beans
- 40g of buckwheat
- 1 tbsp of roughly chopped parsley

Instructions:

- Put the oil over moderate to medium heat in a medium saucepan and fry the onion, carrot, celery, garlic, chili and herbs gently until the onion is soft but not cooked.

- Stir in stock, tomatoes and purée tomatoes and bring to boil. Attach the beans and allow to cook for 30 minutes.

- Add the kale and cook for another 5–10 minutes, then add the parsley, until soft.

- In the meantime, cook the buckwheat as instructed by the package, drain and then serve with stew.

69. SALMON SIRT SUPER SALAD

Makes 1

Ingredients:

- 50g of chicory leaves

- 50g of rocket

- 80g avocado, peeled, stoned and sliced

- 100g of smoked salmon slices (you can also use lentils, cooked chicken breast or tinned tuna)

- 20g red onion, sliced

- 40g celery, sliced

- 1 tbs of capers

- 15g of walnuts, chopped

- 1 tbs of extra-virgin olive oil

- 1 large Medjool date, pitted and chopped

- 10g of parsley, chopped

- Juice ¼ lemon

- 10g of lovage or celery leaves, chopped

Instruction:

- Set the salad sheets on a big dish. Mix all the remaining ingredients and serve over the leaves.

SIMPLE EXERCISES TO MAXIMIZE FAT LOSS

1. WALKING

Walking is one of the strongest weight reduction exercises – and understandably so. For beginners, it is comfortable and simple to continue training without getting stressed or needing to purchase equipment. That is often a smaller-impact workout, which ensures that the joints are not strained.

Harvard's Health reports about 167 calories per 30 minute of walk at a reasonable speed of 4 miles / h are burned by a person of around 155 pounds (70 kg). According to Harvard Health, a 12-week research of 20 women with obesity showed that average weight and waist circumference declined by 1.5 percent and 1.1 inches (2.8 centimeters), respectively, 3 times weekly over the span of 50-70 minutes.

Walking as your everyday routine is easy. Start cycling, using the stairs or getting the dog on extra walks to bring further activity to the day. To continue, consider walking 3–4 days a week for 30 minutes. You may increase the walking time or pace slowly as you need.

2. JOGGING OR RUNNING

Running and jogging are perfect exercises to help you shed weight. While similar, the key difference is that the jog speed is generally between 4 and 6 miles / h (6.4–9.7 miles / h), while the running speed is more than 6 miles per minute (9.7 miles / h).

Health Harvard estimates that a person in 155 pounds (70 kg) burns at a rate of 5 km / h, of about 298 calories per 30 minutes, or 372 calories per thirty minutes at a rate of 6 km / h , respectively, or 9.7 kilometers per hour.

However, experiments have found that jogging and running can effectively incorporate harmful abdominal fat, generally referred to as belly fat. This form of fat surrounds the inner organs and is related to multiple chronic conditions such as cardiac failure and diabetes.

Jogging and cycling are fun activities that are easy to incorporate into your everyday schedule. You can do that anywhere. To start, try

jogging 3–4 days a week for 20–30 minutes. Try to exercise on weaker surfaces such as grass, when you find it difficult to jog or run outdoors. Many treadmills do have an external pad, which will keep the joints smoother.

3. CYCLING

Cycling is a common workout that will help you lose weight and improve health. While outdoor cycling is historically practiced, many fitness centers and gyms offer stationary bikes that allow you to ride when indoor.

Harvard Health has estimated that a person who has a body of 155 pounds (70-kg) burns approx. 260 calories for 30 minutes of a bike ride, at a stationary speed or at a moderate speed of about 12–13,9 mph (19–22,4 km / h) for 30 minutes in a bicycle.

Cycling is not only beneficial for weight reduction, but tests have shown that cyclists are consistently healthier than people that do not routinely bike, have an improved insulin intake and a reduced risk of heart failure, cancer and death.

Cycling is great for people from beginners to athletes at all levels of fitness. Moreover, it is a weightless and low-impact exercise, so your joints will not be stressed much.

4. WEIGHT TRAINING

For people who enjoy losing weight, weight lifting is a common alternative. It is calculated that a person of 155 pounds (70 kg) consumes around 112 calories per weight lifting for 30 minutes, according to Harvard Health.

Weight lifting will also help develop confidence and promote muscle development that will raise your resting metabolic rate (RMR), or reduce the number of calories that the body claims.

A six month research found that the overall metabolic rate was up by 7.4% despite 11 minutes of force-based workouts 3 days a week. This rise was equivalent to a further 125 calories burned every day in this analysis.

The research showed a 9 percent rise in metabolic levels among people contributed to the 24 weeks of weight exercise, which correlated to around 140 more calories a day being consumed. The metabolism growth rate for women amounted to almost 4%, or 50 more calories a day.

Moreover, numerous studies have shown that, compared to aerobics, the body continues to burn calories several hours after training in weight.

5. INTERVAL TRAINING

Interval training (HIIT) is a common concept referring to brief bursts of vigorous workout combined with rest times and is also referred to as high intensity interval training (HIIT).

A HIIT workout usually takes 10-30 minutes, and several calories may be consumed. One research in 9 healthy men showed that HIIT burned between 25 and 30% more calories per minute, including weight training and running on a treadmill, than other workouts.

This means that HIIT can help you burn more calories while you spend less time.

In addition, various studies indicate that HIIT is highly effective in combustion with several chronic conditions, which is consistent with belly fat. HIIT is simple to add into your workout. If you drive, walk, or ride, and pick your workout and your rest periods. All you have to do is select a lesson.

For e.g., a 30-second push, accompanied by a 1-2 minute pedaling, is as hard as you can go on a bike. Repeat 10–30 minutes of this sequence.

6. SWIMMING

Swimming is a fun form of weight reduction and appearance. Harvard Health reports the burning of about 233 calories per half-hours of swimming by a person with 155 pounds (70 kg).

The number of calories that you consume tends to influence how you swim. An individual who burns 298 calories with backstroke, 372 calories with breast-stroke, 409 calories with butterfly stroke and 372 calories water, absorbs 155 pounds every 30 minutes and absorbs 372 calories.

A 12-Week study with 24 mid-aged women showed that body fat, greater flexibility and several risk factors for heart disease, including high total cholesterol and blood triglyceride, were significantly lowered for 60 minutes in 3-fold per week.

The low pressure aspect of the swimming is also an asset that keeps the joints safer. To those with cuts or joint discomfort, it is also a perfect choice.

7. YOGA

Yoga is a common form of stress relief. While not widely regarded as a weight losing workout, it consumes a fair deal of calories and has several other health benefits that may promote weight loss.

Harvard Health reports that an individual of 155 pounds (70 kg) burn around 149 calories per 30 minutes of yoga practice. In a 12-week analysis of 60 obese women , the average waist circumference decreased among all who enrolled in 90-minute yoga sessions a week was 1.5 inches (3.8 cm) in the control group.

Furthermore, emotional and physical health gets strengthened in the Yoga community. Apart from calories burning, study has shown you that yoga will help you to tolerate nutritious food, to regulate over intake and to properly recognize the signs of malnutrition in your body.

Many exercise centers provide yoga courses everywhere. This involves the privacy of your own house, as several direct tutorials are accessible online.

8. PILATES

Pilates is a perfect beginning routine to help you drop weight. A research by the United States Council on Exercise shows that an individual weighing about 140 kg (64 kg) will consume 108 calories in a Pilates beginning class of 30 minutes, or 168 in a high school of the same length.

While Pilates does not eat as many calories as aerobics, many people consider it fun to stick with over time. An 8-week research of 37 middle-aged women showed that Pilates sessions for 90 minutes decreased the neck, stomach and hip diameter substantially 3 times a week in contrast to a control group who did not exercise over the same era.

In addition to reducing weight, Pilates has proven that it decreases lower back discomfort and increases strength, coordination, stability, stamina and physical health.

Seek integrating this into your weekly schedule if you choose to give Pilates a try. In your own house, you can do Pilates or one of Pilates' several gyms.

Combine that with a balanced diet or other workout, including yoga and weight lifting, to help improve weight reduction through Pilates.

What weight do you hope to lose realistically?

The amount of considerations depends on the weight to lose while exercising.

Including:

- **Starting weight.** Those weighing more appear to lose more pounds than those with lesser weight. Nonetheless, the body weight proportion loss is close.

- **Age.** Older individuals continue to bear more weight and lower muscle density, increasing the RMR or the amount of calories the body consumes. A lower RMR can make losing weight harder.

- **Gender.** The fat-to-muscle ratio is higher for men, which can affect the RMR. As a result, even if men eat a similar number of calories they usually lose weight faster than women.

- **Diet.** If you consume more calories than you ingest, weight loss happens. A calorie deficiency is thus important for weight loss.

- **Sleep.** Studies have shown that a lack of sleep will slow down the pace of weight loss and even raise the desire for unsanitary food.

- **Medical conditions.** Medical conditions such as depression and hypothyroidism may slow down weight.

- **Genetics.** Studies also identified a hereditary aspect of weight reduction that may impact many persons with obesity.

Although most individuals choose to lose weight quickly, doctors also suggest that they drop one to 3 pounds a week (0.5-1.36 kg) or around 1% of their body weight.

Dropping weight too quickly can have adverse health consequences. For example, muscle failure may contribute to increased risk of conditions such as gallstones, exhaustion, weakness, starvation, vomiting, irritability, stubbornness, lack of hair and erratic periods.

Moreover, individuals who can so easily drop weight are more likely to rebound. This is important to bear in mind that loss of weight is not a straightforward method so when you first start, it is normal for you to get weight loss quicker.

CONCLUSION

The Sirtfood Diet is the latest diet to take the Planet by storm, developed by the nutritionists Aidan Goggins and Glen Matten. The founders say it is acting to trigger the 'Skinny Genes' in the body. The diet is a dual strategy, concentrating on increasing the body's absorption of products with strong sirtuins and on reducing calories.

Michele states that the advent of the study has also shown that proteins can help to control metabolism, increase muscle quality and boost burn fat. Sirtfoods are also especially rich in polyphenols, as Mikhole describes that they are antioxidant filled micronutrients that have shown themselves to be abundant in polyphenols.

The program is supposed to be followed by participants in order to continue a diet for 2 weeks with a decreased intake and use of 'Sirtfood green juice'. "In the first week, the intake of calories is limited to a thousand calories, with three green juices of Sirt foods and one meal that is high in Sirt food every day," expresses Michele. "You increase your intake of 1500 calories a day the following week by eating two meals rich in Sirt food and two green juices."

There is no particular diet in the long term, but a high Sirt food eating schedule with the addition of green juices is recommended. The makers of the diet say that your diet can result in quick weight loss while preserving your muscle and energy and shielding you from chronic conditions.

Do Not Go Yet; One Last Thing To Do

If you enjoyed this book or found it useful, I'd be very grateful if you'd post a short review on Amazon. Your support does make a difference, and I read all the reviews personally so I can get your feedback and make this book even better.

Thank you so much for your assistance and help!